STUDENT SOLUTIONS MANUAL

John P. Holcomb, Jr.
Cleveland State University

EIGHTH EDITION

BIOSTATISTICS

A Foundation for Analysis in the Health Sciences

Wayne W. Daniel
Georgia State University

WILEY

JOHN WILEY & SONS, INC.

To order books or for customer service, please call 1-800-CALL-WILEY (225-5945).

ISBN-13   978-0-471-70148-4
ISBN-10   0-471-70148-3

Printed in the United States of America.

10 9 8 7 6 5 4 3 2

Printed and bound by Malloy Lithographing, Inc.

Table of Contents

Chapter 2

2.3.1. (a)

Class interval	Frequency	Cumulative frequency	Relative frequency	Cumulative relative frequency
0-0.49	3	3	3.33	3.33
.5-0.99	3	6	3.33	6.67
1.0-1.49	15	21	16.67	23.33
1.5-1.99	15	36	16.67	40.0
2.0-2.49	45	81	50.0	90.00
2.5-2.99	9	90	10.0	100.0

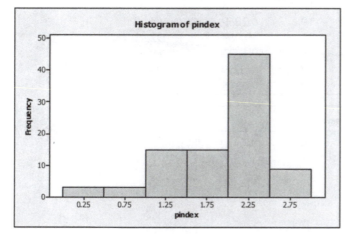

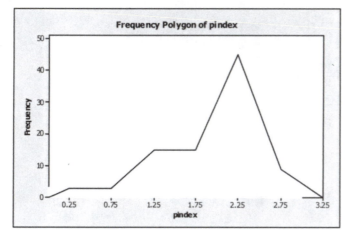

(b)   40.0 %   **(c)** .7667   **(d)** 16.67 %   **(e)** 9   **(f)** 16.67 %

(g)   2.17, because it composes almost 25 percent of the data and is the most frequently occurring value in the data set

(h)   Skewed to the left

2.3.3. (a)

Class interval	Frequency	Cumulative frequency	Relative frequency	Cumulative relative frequency
20-24.99	2	2	0.069	6.9
25-29.99	11	13	0.3793	44.83
30-34.99	6	19	0.2069	65.52
35-39.99	2	21	0.069	72.41
40-44.99	5	26	0.1724	89.66
45-49.99	2	28	0.069	96.55
50-54.99	1	29	0.0345	100

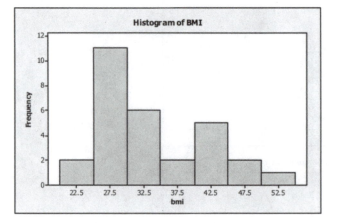

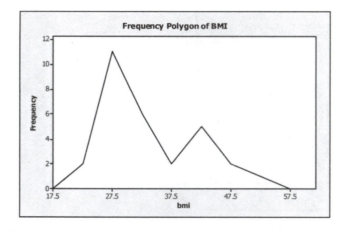

(b) 44.83 % **(c)** 24.14 % **(d)** 34.48 % **(e)** Skewed to the right

(f) 21

2.3.5. (a)

Class interval	Frequency	Relative frequency
0-2	5	0.1111
3-5	16	0.3556
6-8	13	0.2889
9-11	5	0.1111
12-14	4	0.0889
15-17	2	0.0444
	45	1.000

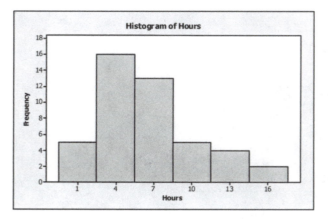

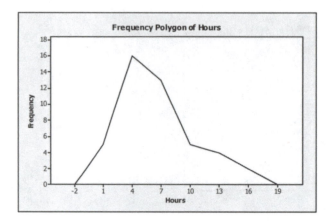

(b) Skewed to the right

2.3.7. (a)

Class interval	Frequency	Cumulative frequency	Relative frequency	Cumulative relative frequency
110-139	8	8	0.0516	0.0516
140-169	16	24	0.1032	0.1548
170-199	46	70	0.2968	0.4516
200-229	49	119	0.3161	0.7677
230-259	26	145	0.1677	0.9355
260-289	9	154	0.581	0.9935
290-319	1	155	0.065	1.0000

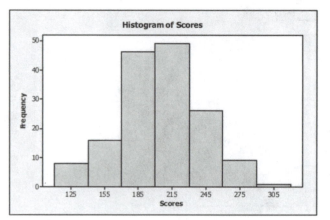

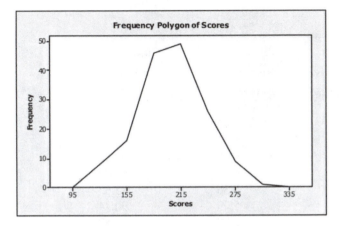

(b) Not greatly skewed

2.3.9. (a)

Stem-and-leaf display: Hospital A	Stem-and-leaf display: Hospital B
Stem-and-leaf of C1 N = 25 Leaf Unit = 1.0	Stem-and-leaf of C2 N = 25 Leaf Unit = 1.0

```
    1    17 1                          1    12 5
    2    18 4                          2    13 5
    4    19 15                         4    14 35
    9    20 11259                      9    15 02445
   (6)   21 233447                    (4)   16 5678
   10    22 2259                      12    17 38
    6    23 389                       10    18 466
    3    24 589                        7    19 0059
                                       3    20 3
                                       2    21 24
```

(b) Both asymmetric, A is skewed left and B is skewed right

5

2.3.11. (a)

Class interval	Frequency	Cumulative frequency	Relative frequency	Cumulative relative frequency
.0-.0999	45	45	20.83	20.83
.1-.1999	50	95	23.15	43.98
.2-.2999	34	129	15.74	59.72
.3-.3999	21	150	9.72	69.44
.4-.4999	23	173	10.65	80.09
.5-.5999	12	185	5.56	85.65
.6-.6999	11	196	5.09	90.74
.7-.7999	6	202	2.78	93.52
.8-.8999	4	206	1.85	95.37
.9-.9999	5	211	2.31	97.69
1.0-1.0999	4	215	1.85	99.54
1.1-1.1999	1	216	0.46	100.00

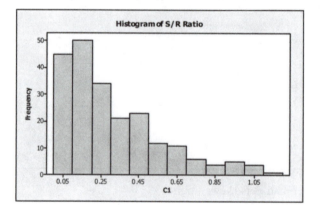

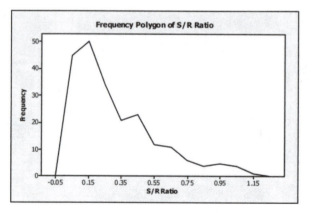

```
Stem-and-leaf of C1        N  = 216
Leaf Unit = 0.010

   46      0  12455667788889999999999999999999999999999999
   96      1  0000000000112223333444455555566666667777777778888999
  (34)     2  0011111223444444445566666788889999
   86      3  001111244445556668999
   65      4  00001122223333444568899
   42      5  002334444599
   30      6  02236788999
   19      7  012289
   13      8  0237
    9      9  05588
    4     10  236
    1     11  6
```

(b) Skewed right **(c)** 10, 4.62 % **(d)** 196, 90.74 %; 67, 31.02 %, 143, 19.91 %

2.5.1.

Mean	Median	Mode	Range
193.6	205.0	no mode	255

Variance	Standard Deviation	Coefficient of Variation	IQR
5568.14	74.62	38.53	100.5

The median is a better measure of center because the data is skewed left.

2.5.3.

Mean	Median	Mode	Range
47.42	46.35	54.0, 33.0	29.6

Variance	Standard Deviation	Coefficient of Variation	IQR
76.56	8.75	18.45	13.72

Either the mean or median is a good measure of center.

2.5.5.

Mean	Median	Mode	Range
16.75	15	15	43

Variance	Standard Deviation	Coefficient of Variation	IQR
124.10	11.14	66.51	8.25

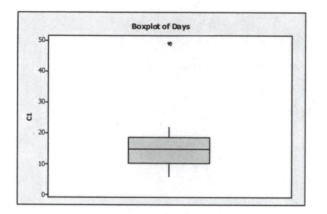

The median is a better measure of center because it is not influenced by the outlier.

2.5.7.

Mean	**Median**	**Mode**	**Range**
1.8172	2	2.17	2.83

Variance	**Standard Deviation**	**Coefficient of Variation**	**IQR**
.3164	.5625	30.96	.6700

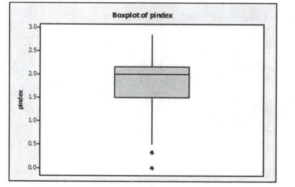

The median is a better measure of center because the distribution is left skewed.

2.5.9.

Mean	**Median**	**Mode**	**Range**
33.87	30.49	none	29.84

Variance	**Standard Deviation**	**Coefficient of Variation**	**IQR**
64.00	8.00	23.62	13.4

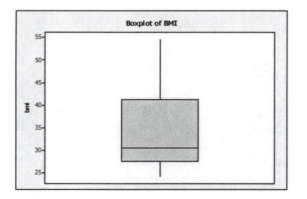

The median is a better measure of center because the distribution is right skewed.

2.5.11.

Mean	Median	Mode	Range
6.711	7.00	7.00	16

Variance	Standard Deviation	Coefficient of Variation	IQR
16.21	4.026	59.99	5.5

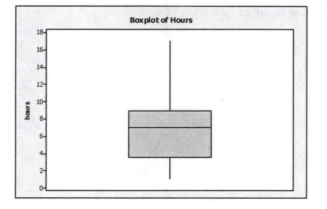

The median is a better measure of center because the distribution is slightly right skewed.

2.5.13.

Mean	Median	Mode	Range
204.19	204	212, 198	196

Variance	Standard Deviation	Coefficient of Variation	IQR
1258.12	35.47	17.37	46

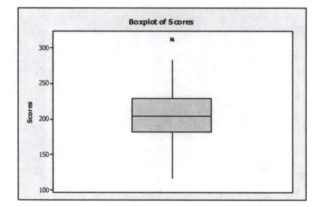

Either the mean or median is a good measure of center.

Chapter 2 Review Exercises

13.
(a) Leaf Unit = 1.0

```
   2      2 55
   4      2 67
   7      2 999
  10      3 001
  17      3 2223333
 (12)     3 444555555555
  21      3 6666666666666666666677
```

(b)   skewed   **(c)** 37 weeks is considered full-term, surgery is done before birth

(d) $\bar{x} = 33.680$, median $= 35.00$, $s^2 = 10.304$, $s = 3.210$

15. $\bar{x} = 43.39$, median = 42, $s = 17.09$, C.V. = 39.387

(b)
Stem-and-leaf of GFR   N = 28
Leaf Unit = 1.0

```
    1     1 8
    6     2 11377
   12     3 022267
   (7)    4 1223388
    9     5 158
    6     6 02378
    1     7
    1     8 8
```

(c)

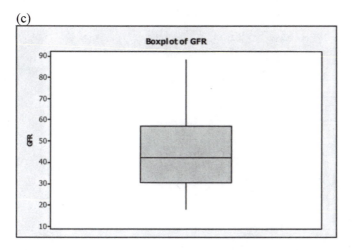

(d) 67.9 %, 96.55 %, 100 %

19. $\bar{x} = 3.95$, Median = 3, $s^2 = 12.998$, $s = 3.605$

27.

Variable	N	Mean	SE Mean	StDev	Minimum	Q1	Median	Q3	Maximum
C1	216	0.3197	0.0169	0.2486	0.0269	0.1090	0.2440	0.4368	1.1600

Variance = .0681, IQR = .3277, Range = 1.1331, IQR/R = .2892

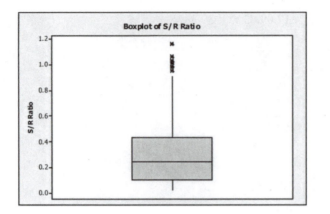

29. (a)

Variable	N	Mean	Median	TrMean	StDev	SE Mean
nutri	107	75.40	73.80	74.77	13.64	1.32

Variable	Minimum	Maximum	Q1	Q3
nutri	45.60	130.00	67.50	80.60

Variance = 186.0496, Range = 84.4, IQR = 13.1 IQR/R = .1552

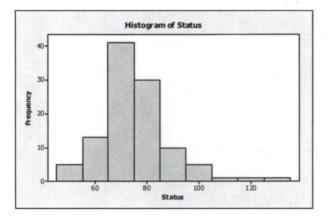

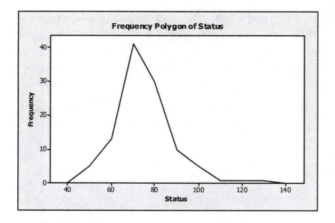

```
Stem-and-leaf of C1        N  = 107
Leaf Unit = 1.0

     1     4 5
     5     5 0004
    12     5 5556899
    18     6 013444
    31     6 5555666777888
   (28)    7 0000011122222222333333344444
    48     7 666666666677888999
    30     8 000002234444
    18     8 56889
    13     9 01223
     8     9 679
     5    10 00
     3    10 9
     2    11
     2    11
     2    12 3
     1    12
     1    13 0
```

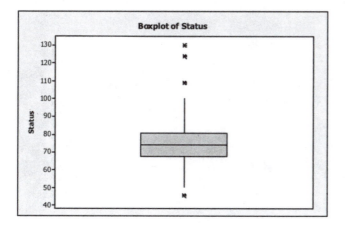

(d) 75.4 ± 13.64 gives endpoints 61.76 and 89.04. There are 79 points within one standard deviation giving $79/107 = .7383$ or 74% within one s.d. of the mean.

$75.4 \pm 2(13.64)$ gives endpoints 48.12 and 102.68. There 103 points within 2 s.d.'s of the mean giving $103/107 = .9626$ or 96% within two s.d.'s of the mean.

$75.4 \pm 3(13.64)$ gives endpoints 34.48 and 116.32. There are 105 points within 3 s.d.'s of the mean giving $105/107 = .9813$ or 98% within three s.d.'s of the mean.

(e) $102/107 = .9533$ **(f)** $1/107 = .0093$

Chapter 3

3.4.1.
(a) $P(\text{Woman}) = 679/1024 = .6631$

(b)   Marginal probability

(c)   Using the definition of marginal probability:
$P(\text{Woman}) = P(\text{Woman} \cap \text{No Victimization}) + P(\text{Woman} \cap \text{Partner}) +$
$P(\text{Woman} \cap \text{Nonpartners}) + P(\text{Woman} \cap \text{Multiple Victimization}) = 611/1024 +$
$34/1024 + 16/1024 + 18/1024 = .5967 + .0332 + .0156 + .0176 = .6631.$
The compliment rule: $P(\text{Woman}) = 1 - P(\text{Man}) = 1 - 345/1024 = 1 - .3369 = .6631$

(d) $34/1024 = .0332$ **(e)** Joint probability   **(f)** $17/345 = .0493$

(g)   Conditional probability

(h) $(345/1024) + (44/1024) - (10/1024) = .3369 + .0430 - .0098 = .3701$

(i)   Addition rule

3.4.3.
(a) $P(\text{Male} \cap \text{Split drugs}) = 349/1021 = .3418$

(b) $P(\text{Male or Split drugs or both}) =$
$(673/1021) + (569/1021) - (349/1021) = .6592 + .5573 - .3418 = .8747$

(c) $P(\text{Male} \mid \text{Split drugs}) = 349/569 = .6134$ **(d)** $P(\text{Male}) = 673/1021 = .6592$

3.4.5. $1 - .05 = .95$

3.4.7. $P(\text{H}) = .35, P(\text{S}|\text{H}) = .86, P(\text{S} \cap \text{H}) = P(\text{H})*P(\text{S}|\text{H}) = (.35)(.86) = .301$

3.5.1.
(a)   A subject having the symptom(S) and not having the disease.

(b)   A subject not having S but having the disease.

(c) $P(\text{S}|\text{D}) = 744/775 = .96$

(d) $P(\overline{S} \mid \overline{D}) = 1359/1380 = .9848$

(e) $P(S \mid \overline{D}) = 21/1380 = .0152; P(D \mid S) = (.96)(.001)/[(.96)(.001) + (.0152)(.999)] = .0595$

(f) $P(\overline{S} \mid D) = 31/775 = .04; P(\overline{D} \mid \overline{S}) = (.9848)(.999)/[(.9848)(.999) + (.04)(.001)] = .99996$

(g)

$$P(D \mid S) = \frac{(.96)(.0001)}{(.96)(.0001) + (.0152)(.9999)} = .00628$$

$$P(\overline{D} \mid \overline{S}) = \frac{(.9848)(.9999)}{(.9848)(.9999) + (.04)(.0001)} = .999996$$

$$P(D \mid S) = \frac{(.96)(.01)}{(.96)(.01) + (.0152)(.99)} = .3895$$

$$P(\overline{D} \mid \overline{S}) = \frac{(.9848)(.99)}{(.9848)(.99) + (.04)(.01)} = .9996$$

$$P(D \mid S) = \frac{(.96)(.10)}{(.96)(.10) + (.0152)(.90)} = .8753$$

$$P(\overline{D} \mid \overline{S}) = \frac{(.9848)(.90)}{(.9848)(.90) + (.04)(.10)} = .9955$$

3.5.3. Sensitivity $= P(T \mid D) = .927$; Specificity $= P(\overline{T} \mid \overline{D}) = .997$;

$P(D) = 1/320000 = .00003125$; $P(\overline{D}) = 1 - .00003125 = .99996875$

$P(\overline{T} \mid D) = 1 - P(T \mid D) = 1 - .927 = .073$

Predictive Value Negative $= \dfrac{(.997)(.99996875)}{(.997)(.99996875) + (.073)(.00003125)} = .99999977$

Chapter 3 Review Exercises

3.
(a) $459/2142 = .2143$ **(b)** $319/578 = .5519$ **(c)** $329/2142 = .1536$

(d) $578/2142 + 490/2142 - 88/2142 = .2698 + .2288 - .0411 = .4575$

(e) $1 - (1057/2142) = .5065$

5.
(a) $17/126 = .1349$ **(b)** $52/126 + 42/126 - 17/126 = .4127 + .3333 - .1349 = .6111$

(c) $42/126 = .3333$ **(d)** $1 - (52/126) = .5873$ **(e)** $15/42 = .3571$

(f) $1 - (42/126) = .6667$ **(g)** 0 (These are mutually exclusive events)

(h) $17/52 = .3269$

7.
(a)

1. $\dfrac{220}{1000} = .2200$ **2.** $\dfrac{500}{1000} = .5000$ **3.** $\dfrac{55}{1000} = .0555$

4. $\dfrac{55}{500} = .1100$ **5.** $\dfrac{390}{1000} + \dfrac{500}{1000} - \dfrac{300}{1000} = .5900$

(b)

1. $\dfrac{300}{1000} = .3000$ **2.** $\dfrac{390}{1000} = .3900$ **3.** $\dfrac{390}{1000} = .3900$

4. $\dfrac{65}{390} = .1667$ **5.** $\dfrac{70}{1000} = .0700$ **6.** $\dfrac{300}{500} = .6000$

9.
(a) $5235/121196 = .0432$ **(b)** $3102/121196 = .0256$ **(c)** $2992/121196 = .0247$

(d) $2991/3103 = .9639$ **(e)** $2991/5235 = .5713$

(f)   Sensitivity $= P(T \mid D) = P(A \mid B)\,2991/3103.9639$

(g)   Specificity $= P(\overline{T} \mid \overline{D}) = P(\overline{A} \mid \overline{B}) = 115849/118093 = .9810$

11. $(.03)(.20) = .0060$

13.

Disease?	Symptom		Total
	Y	N	
Y	.18	.05	.23
N	.02	.75	.77
Total	.20	.80	1.00

$P(D \mid \overline{S}) = .05/.8 = .0625$

15.   Mothers 24 years of age or younger

17. $P(G) = 0$, since A and B are mutually exclusive. A mother cannot be both under 20 and between 20 and 24 years of age.

19.

(a) Plasma lipoprotein levels between 10 and 15 <u>or</u> greater than or equal to 30.

(b) Plasma lipoprotein levels between 10 and 15 <u>and</u> greater than or equal to 30.

(c) Plasma lipoprotein levels between 10 and 15 <u>and</u> less than or equal to 20.

(d) Plasma lipoprotein levels between 10 and 15 <u>or</u> less than or equal to 20.

21.

(a) Sensitivity $= P(T \mid D) = 214/287 = .7456$

(b) Specificity $= P(\overline{T} \mid \overline{D}) = 330/1000 = .3300$

23. $P(T \mid \overline{D}) = 1 - \text{specificity} = 1 - .85 = .15; \ P(D \mid T) = \dfrac{(.95)(.002)}{(.95)(.002) + (.15)(1 - .002)} = .0125$

Chapter 4

4.3.1.

(a) $\quad _{20}C_3(.76)^{17}(.24)^3 = .1484$

(b) $\quad 1 - \left[_{20}C_0(.76)^{20}(.24)^0 + _{20}C_1(.76)^{19}(.24)^1 + _{20}C_2(.76)^{18}(.24)^2 \right] =$

$1 - [.0041 + .0261 + .0783] = .8915$

(c) $\quad _{20}C_0(.76)^{20}(.24)^0 + _{20}C_1(.76)^{19}(.24)^1 + _{20}C_2(.76)^{18}(.24)^2 = .0041 + .0261 + .0783 =$

$.1085$

(d) $\quad _{20}C_3(.76)^{17}(.24)^3 + _{20}C_4(.76)^{16}(.24)^4 +$

$_{20}C_5(.76)^{15}(.24)^5 + _{20}C_6(.76)^{14}(.24)^6 + _{20}C_7(.76)^{13}(.24)^7 =$
$.1484 + .1991 + .2012 + .1589 + .1003 = .8079$

4.3.3.

(a) $\quad _5C_0(.76)^5(.24)^0 = .2536$

(b) $\quad _5C_2(.76)^3(.24)^2 + _5C_3(.76)^2(.24)^3 + _5C_4(.76)(.24)^4 + _5C_5(.76)^0(.24)^5 =$
$.2529 + .0798 + .0126 + .0008 = .3461$

(c) $\quad _5C_1(.76)^4(.24)^1 + _5C_2(.76)^3(.24)^2 + _5C_3(.76)^2(.24)^3 =$
$.4003 + .2529 + .0798 = .7330$

(d) $\quad _5C_0(.76)^5(.24)^0 + _5C_1(.76)^4(.24)^1 + _5C_2(.76)^3(.24)^2 =$
$.2536 + .4003 + .2529 = .9068$

(e) $\quad _5C_5(.76)^0(.24)^5 = .0008$

4.3.5. $\quad \mu = np = 15(.32) = 4.8; \sigma^2 = npq = 15(.32)(.68) = 3.264$

4.3.7.

(a) $\;_3C_0(.81)^3(.19)^0 = .5314$ **(b)** $\;_3C_1(.81)^2(.19)^1 = .3740$

(c) $\;_3C_2(.81)^1(.19)^2 +\;_3C_3(.81)^0(.19)^3 = .0877 + .0069 = .0946$

(d) $1 -\;_3C_3(.81)^0(.19)^3 = 1 - .0069 = .9931$

(e) $\;_3C_2(.81)^1(.19)^2 +\;_3C_3(.81)^0(.19)^3 = .0877 + .0069 = .0946$

(f) $\;_3C_3(.81)^0(.19)^3 = .0069$

4.3.9.

Number of Successes, x	Probability, $f(x)$
0	$_3C_0(.2)^3(.8)^0 = .008$
1	$_3C_1(.2)^2(.8)^1 = .096$
2	$_3C_2(.2)^1(.8)^2 = .384$
3	$_3C_3(.2)^0(.8)^3 = .512$
Total	1.000

4.4.1.

(a) $\dfrac{e^{-4}4^5}{5!} = .156$

(b) $1 - \left[\dfrac{e^{-4}4^0}{0!} + \dfrac{e^{-4}4^1}{1!} + \dfrac{e^{-4}4^2}{2!} + \dfrac{e^{-4}4^3}{3!} + \dfrac{e^{-4}4^4}{4!} + \dfrac{e^{-4}4^5}{5!} \right] = 1 - .785 = .215$

(c) $\dfrac{e^{-4}4^0}{0!} + \dfrac{e^{-4}4^1}{1!} + \dfrac{e^{-4}4^2}{2!} + \dfrac{e^{-4}4^3}{3!} + \dfrac{e^{-4}4^4}{4!} = .629$

(d) $\dfrac{e^{-4}4^5}{5!} + \dfrac{e^{-4}4^6}{6!} + \dfrac{e^{-4}4^7}{7!} = .156 + .104 + .060 = .320$

4.4.3.

(a) $\dfrac{e^{-5}5^7}{7!} = .105$ **(b)** $1-.968 = .032$ **(c)** $\dfrac{e^{-5}5^0}{0!} = .007$

(d) $\dfrac{e^{-5}5^0}{0!} + \dfrac{e^{-5}5^1}{1!} + \dfrac{e^{-5}5^2}{2!} + \dfrac{e^{-5}5^3}{3!} + \dfrac{e^{-5}5^4}{4!} = .440$

4.4.5.

(a) $.252-.166 = .086$ **(b)** $1 - .054 = .946$ **(c)** $.463$

(d) $.764-.100 = .664$ **(e)** $.026$

4.6.1. $P(0 \le z \le 1.43) = .9236 - .5 = .4236$

4.6.3. $P(z = .55) = 0, \ \ P(z \ge .55) = 1 - .7088 = .2912$

4.6.5. $P(z < -2.33) = .0099$

4.6.7. $P(-1.96 \le z \le 1.96) = .975 - .025 = .95$

4.6.9. $P(-1.65 \le z \le 1.65) = .9505 - .0495 = .901$

4.6.11.

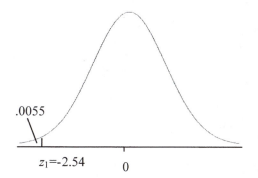

.0055

$z_1 = -2.54$ 0

4.6.13.

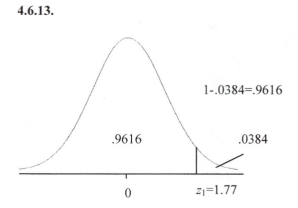

1-.0384=.9616

.9616   .0384

0   z_1=1.77

4.6.15.

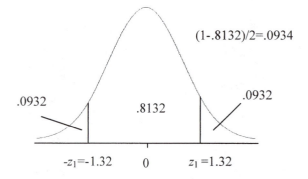

(1-.8132)/2=.0934

.0932   .0932

.8132

$-z_1$=-1.32   0 z_1 =1.32

4.7.1.

(a) $P(600 \leq x \leq 1000) = P\left(\dfrac{600-870}{211} \leq z \leq \dfrac{1000-870}{211} \right)$

   $= P(-1.28 \leq z \leq .62) = .7324 - .1003 = .6321$

(b) $P(x > 900) = P\left(z > \dfrac{900-870}{211} \right) = P(z > .14) = 1 - .5557 = .4443$

(c) $P(x < 500) = P\left(z < \dfrac{500-870}{211} \right) = P(z < -1.75) = .0401$

(d) $P(900 \leq x \leq 1100) = P\left(\dfrac{900-870}{211} \leq z \leq \dfrac{1100-870}{211} \right)$

   $= P(.14 \leq z \leq 1.09) = .8621 - .5557 = .3064$

4.7.3.

(a) $P(x < 15) = P\left(z < \dfrac{15 - 30.23}{13.84}\right) = P(z < -1.10) = .1357$

(b) $P(x > 40) = P\left(z > \dfrac{40 - 30.23}{13.84}\right) = P(z > .71) = .1 - .7611 = .2389$

(c) $P(14 \le x \le 50) = P\left(\dfrac{14 - 30.23}{13.84} \le z \le \dfrac{40 - 30.23}{13.84}\right)$

$= P(-1.17 \le z \le .71) = .7611 - .1210 = .6401$

(d) $P(x < 10) = P\left(z < \dfrac{10 - 30.23}{13.84}\right) = P(z < -1.46) = .0721$

(e) $P(10 \le x \le 20) = P\left(\dfrac{10 - 30.23}{13.84} \le z \le \dfrac{20 - 30.23}{13.84}\right)$

$= P(-1.46 \le z \le -.74) = .2296 - .0721 = .1575$

4.7.5.

(a) $P(180 < x < 200) = P\left(\dfrac{180 - 200}{20} < z < \dfrac{200 - 200}{20}\right) = P(-1 < z < 0) = .3413$

(b) $P(x > 225) = P\left(z > \dfrac{225 - 200}{20}\right) = P(z > 1.25) = 1 - .9844 = .1056$

(c) $P(x < 150) = P\left(z < \dfrac{150 - 200}{20}\right) = P(z < -2.5) = .0062$

(d) $P(190 < x < 210) = P\left(\dfrac{190 - 200}{20} < z < \dfrac{210 - 200}{20}\right) =$

$P(-.5 < z < .5) = .6915 - .3085 = .3830$

4.7.7.

(a) $P(x > 155) = P\left(z > \dfrac{155 - 132}{15}\right) = P(z > 1.53) = 1 - .9370 = .0630$

(b) $P(x \le 100) = P\left(z < \dfrac{100 - 132}{15}\right) = P(z \le -2.13) = .0166$

(c) $P(105 < x < 145) = P\left(\dfrac{105 - 132}{15} < z < \dfrac{145 - 132}{15}\right) =$

$P(-1.8 < z < .87) = .8078 - .0359 = .7719$

Chapter 4 Review Exercises

15. (a) $_{10}C_7 .65^3 .35^7 = .0212$ **(b)** $1 - .9051 = .0949$ **(c)** $_{10}C_0 .65^{10} .35^0 = .0135$

(d) $.9740 - .2616 = .7124$

17.
(a) $.077 - .043 = .034$ **(b)** $.467 - .000 = .467$ **(c)** $1 - .077 = .923$

(d) $.010$ **(e)** $.127 - .022 = .105$

19. (a) $1 - .5033 = .4967$ **(b)** $.5033$ **(c)** $.1678$

(d) $1 - .9896 = .0104$ **(e)** $.9896 - .1678 = .8218$

21.

(a) $P(x > 75) = P\left(z > \dfrac{75 - 60}{10}\right) = P(z > 1.5) = 1 - .9332 = .0668$

(b) $P(55 \le x \le 75) = P\left(\dfrac{55 - 60}{10} z \le \dfrac{75 - 60}{10}\right) =$

$P(-.5 \le z \le 1.5) = .9332 - .3085 = .6247$

(c) $P(50 \le x \le 70) = P\left(\dfrac{50 - 60}{10} z \le \dfrac{70 - 60}{10}\right) = P(-1 \le z \le 1) = .8413 - .1587 = .6826$

23.

(a) $P(x < 200) = P\left(z < \dfrac{200 - 500}{100}\right) = P(z < -3) = .0013 .0013$

(b) $P(x \geq 650) = P\left(z \geq \dfrac{650 - 500}{100}\right) = P(z \geq 1.5) = 1 - .9332 = .0668$

(c) $P(350 \leq x \leq 675) = P\left(\dfrac{350 - 500}{100} \leq z \leq \dfrac{675 - 500}{100}\right)$
$= P(-1.5 \leq z \leq 1.75) = .9599 - .0668 = .8931$

25. $z_0 = \dfrac{x - \mu}{\sigma}; P(z \geq z_0) = .0985; 1 - .0985 = .9015$

$P(z \leq 1.29) = .9015; 1.29 = \dfrac{70 - \mu}{10} \Rightarrow 70 - \mu = 12.90 \Rightarrow \mu = 57.10$

27.

(a) $P(z \leq -2.35) = .0094 \Rightarrow -2.35 = \dfrac{k - 100}{15} \Rightarrow k = 64.75$

(b) $P(z \geq 1.23) = .1093 \Rightarrow 1.23 = \dfrac{k - 100}{15} \Rightarrow k = 118.45$

(c) $P(z \leq 2.01) = .9778 \Rightarrow 2.01 = \dfrac{k - 100}{15} \Rightarrow k = 130.15$

(d) $(1 - .9660)/2 = .0170; .9660 + .0170 = .9830$

$P(z \leq 2.12) = .9830 \Rightarrow 2.12 = \dfrac{k - 100}{15} \Rightarrow k = 131.8$

29. $P(z \leq z_0) = .9904; z_0 = 2.34 \Rightarrow 2.34 = \dfrac{50 - \mu}{15} \Rightarrow \mu = 14.90$

31. $P(z \leq z_0) = .0778; z_0 = -1.42; -1.42 = \dfrac{10 - 25}{\sigma} \Rightarrow \sigma = 10.6$

33.

(a)   Could be Bernoulli if we assume each child has an equal chance of being a boy or girl;

(b)   Not a Bernoulli - More than 2 possible outcomes

(c)   Not a Bernoulli - Weight is a continuous variable

Chapter 5

5.3.1. Sampling distribution mean: 204, Standard Error: $\sigma_{\bar{x}} = \dfrac{\sigma}{\sqrt{n}} = \dfrac{44}{\sqrt{50}} = 6.2225$

5.3.3.

(a) $\sigma_{\bar{x}} = 1/\sqrt{9} = .3333, \quad z = \dfrac{6 - 5.7}{.3333} = .90, \quad P(\bar{x} > 6) = 1 - P(z \le .90) = 1 - .8159 = .1841$

(b) $z_1 = \dfrac{5 - 5.7}{.3333} = -2.10, \quad z_2 = .90$

$P(5 \le \bar{x} \le 6) = P(-2.10 \le z \le .90) = .8159 - .0179 = .7980$

(c) $z = \dfrac{5.2 - 5.7}{.3333} = -1.50, \quad P(\bar{x} < 5.2) = P(z < -1.50) = .0668$

5.3.5.

(a) $\sigma_{\bar{x}} = 1476/\sqrt{75} = 170.4338, \quad z = \dfrac{2450 - 2940}{170.4338} = -2.88$

$P(\bar{x} < 2450) = P(z < -2.88) = .0020$

(b) $z = \dfrac{3100 - 2940}{170.4338} = .94, \quad P(\bar{x} > 3100) = 1 - P(z \le .94) = 1 - .8264 = .1736$

(c) $z_1 = \dfrac{2500 - 2940}{170.4338} = -2.58, \quad z_2 = \dfrac{3300 - 2940}{170.4338} = 2.11$

$P(2500 \le \bar{x} \le 3300) = P(-2.58 \le z \le 2.11) = .9826 - .0049 = .9777$

(d) $z_1 = -2.58, \quad z_2 = \dfrac{2900 - 2940}{170.4338} = -.23$

$P(2500 \le \bar{x} \le 2900) = P(-2.58 \le z \le -.23) = .4090 - .0049 = .4041$

5.3.7. $\sigma_{\bar{x}} = 16/\sqrt{64} = 2$

(a) $P(45 \leq \bar{x} \leq 55) = P\left(\dfrac{45-50}{2} \leq z \leq \dfrac{55-50}{2}\right)$

$= P(-2.5 \leq z \leq 2.5) = .9938 - .0062 = .9876$

(b) $P(\bar{x} > 53) = P\left(z > \dfrac{53-50}{2}\right) = P(z > 1.5) = 1 - .9332 = .0668$

(c) $P(\bar{x} < 47) = P\left(z < \dfrac{47-50}{2}\right) = P(z < -1.5) = .0668$

(d) $P(49 \leq \bar{x} \leq 56) = P\left(\dfrac{49-50}{2} \leq z \leq \dfrac{56-50}{2}\right)$

$= P(-.5 \leq z \leq 3) = .9987 - .3085 = .6902$

5.3.9.

Sample	$\bar{x}$
6, 8, 10	8.00
6, 8, 12	8.67
6, 8, 14	9.33
6, 10 ,12	9.33
6, 10, 14	10.00
6, 12, 14	10.67
8, 10, 12	10.00
8, 10, 14	10.67
8, 12, 14	11.33
10, 12, 14	12.00

$\mu_{\bar{x}} = (8.00 + 8.67 + \cdots + 12.00)/10 = 10$

$\sigma_{\bar{x}}^2 = \dfrac{(8-10)^2 + (8.67-10)^2 + \cdots + (12.00-10)^2}{10} = 1.3333$

5.4.1. $\sigma_{\bar{x}_B - \bar{x}_A} = \sqrt{\dfrac{34.7^2}{50} + \dfrac{37.2^2}{50}} = 7.1943$

$P(\bar{x}_B - \bar{x}_A > 8) = P\left(z > \dfrac{8 - (189 - 183)}{7.1943}\right) = P(z > .28) = 1 - .6103 = .3897$

5.4.3. $\sigma_{\bar{x}_1 - \bar{x}_2} = \sqrt{\dfrac{100}{25} + \dfrac{80}{16}} = 3$

$$P(\bar{x}_1 - \bar{x}_2 \geq 8) = P\left(z \geq \dfrac{8-0}{3}\right) = P(z \geq 2.67) = 1 - .9962 = .0038$$

5.4.5. $P(\bar{x}_G - \bar{x}_B > 10) = P\left(z > \dfrac{10 - (15.6 - 9.7)}{\sqrt{\dfrac{6^2}{40} + \dfrac{9.5^2}{35}}}\right) = P(z > 2.20) = 1 - .9861 = .0139$

5.5.1. $z = \dfrac{.40 - .32}{\sqrt{\dfrac{.32(.68)}{50}}} = 1.21; \quad P(z > 1.21) = 1 - .8869 = .1131$

5.5.3. $z = \dfrac{.70 - .64}{\sqrt{\dfrac{.64(.36)}{125}}} = 1.40; \quad P(z \geq 1.40) = 1 - .9192 = .0808$

5.5.5. $\sigma_{\hat{p}} = \sqrt{\dfrac{(.6)(.4)}{100}} = .0490$

(a) $P(\hat{p} \geq .65) = P\left(z \geq \dfrac{.65 - .6}{.0490}\right) = P(z \geq 1.02) = 1 - .8461 = .1539$

(b) $P(\hat{p} \leq .58) = P\left(z \leq \dfrac{.58 - .6}{.0490}\right) = P(z \leq -.41) = .3409$

(c) $P(.56 \leq \hat{p} \leq .63) = P\left(\dfrac{.56 - .6}{.0490} \leq z \leq \dfrac{.63 - .6}{.0490}\right) =$

$P(-.82 \leq z \leq .61) = .7291 - .2061 = .5230$

5.6.1. $\sigma_{\hat{p}_1 - \hat{p}_2} = \sqrt{\dfrac{(.095)(.905)}{100} + \dfrac{(.049)(.951)}{120}} = .0353$

$$P(\hat{p}_1 - \hat{p}_2 \geq .09) = P\left(z \geq \dfrac{.09 - (.095 - .049)}{.0353}\right) = P(z \geq 1.25) = 1 - .8944 = .1056$$

5.6.3. $\sigma_{\hat{p}_1-\hat{p}_2} = \sqrt{\dfrac{(.21)(.79)}{120}+\dfrac{(.13)(.87)}{130}} = .0475$

$$P(.04 < \hat{p}_1 - \hat{p}_2 < .20) = P\left(\dfrac{.04-.08}{.0475} < z < \dfrac{.20-.08}{.0475}\right) = P(-.84 < z < 2.53) = .9943 - .2005 = .7938$$

Chapter 5 Review Exercises

11. $P(\overline{x} > 25) = P\left(z > \dfrac{25-23.1}{3.7/\sqrt{45}}\right) = P(z > 3.44) = 1 - .9997 = .0003$

13. $\sigma_{\overline{x}_M - \overline{x}_W} = \sqrt{\dfrac{3.3^2}{50}+\dfrac{3.7^2}{45}} = .7225$

$$P(\overline{x}_M - \overline{x}_W > 3) = p\left(z > \dfrac{3-(24.7-23.1)}{.7225}\right) = P(z > 1.94) = 1 - .9738 = .0262$$

15. $P(\overline{x} > 19) = P\left(z > \dfrac{19-17.9}{10.9/\sqrt{120}}\right) = P(z > 1.11) = 1 - .8665 = .1335$

17. $P(\hat{p} > .25) = P\left(z > \dfrac{.25-.19}{\sqrt{\dfrac{(.19)(.81)}{65}}}\right) = P(z > 1.23) = 1 - .8907 = .1093$

19. $P(\hat{p} < .20) = P\left(z < \dfrac{.20-.23}{\sqrt{\dfrac{(.23)(.77)}{250}}}\right) = P(z < -1.13) = .1292$

21. $_{10}C_5 = \dfrac{10!}{5!5!} = 252$

23. $\mu_{\hat{p}} = .53, \ \sigma_{\hat{p}} = \sqrt{(.53)(.47)/110} = .0476$

25. At least approximately normally distributed

27. $P(22 \le \bar{x} \le 29) = P\left(\dfrac{22-25}{1.18} \le z \le \dfrac{29-25}{1.18}\right)$

$= P(-2.54 \le z \le 3.39) = .9997 - .0055 = .9942$

29.

(a) No, since 8(.5) = 4 and 4<5.

(b) Yes, since 30(.4) = 12 and 30(.6) = 18 are both >5.

(c) No, since 30(.1) = 3 is less than 5.

(d) Yes, since 1000(.01) = 10 and 1000(.99)=990 are both greater than 5.

(e) Yes, since 100(.9)=90 and 100(.1) = 10 are both greater than 5.

(f) Yes, since 150(.05)=7.5 and 150(.95) = 142.5 are both greater than 5.

Chapter 6

6.2.1. $\sigma_{\bar{x}} = 10/\sqrt{49} = 1.43$

(a) $90 \pm 1.645(1.43) = (88,92)$ **(b)** $90 \pm 1.96(1.43) = (87,93)$

(c) $90 \pm 2.58(1.43) = (86,94)$

6.2.3. $\sigma_{\bar{x}} = 3/\sqrt{64} = .375$

(a) $8.25 \pm 1.645(.375) = (7.63,8.87)$ **(b)** $8.25 \pm 1.96(.375) = (7.51,8.99)$

(c) $8.25 \pm 2.58(.375) = (7.28,9.22)$

6.2.5. $\bar{x} = 1747.625,\ \sigma_{\bar{x}} = 350/\sqrt{16} = 87.5$

(a) $1747.625 \pm 1.645(87.5) = (1603.688,1891.563)$

(b) $1747.625 \pm 1.96(87.5) = (1576.125,1919.125)$

(c) $1747.625 \pm 2.58(87.5) = (1521.875,1973.375)$

6.3.1.

(a) 2.1448 **(b)** 2.8073 **(c)** 1.8946 **(d)** 2.0452

6.3.3.

(a) $(.4)(\sqrt{15}) = 1.549;\ (.1)(\sqrt{15}) = .387$

(b) $3.5 \pm 2.1448(.4) = (2.64,4.36);\ .7 \pm 2.1448(.1) = (.49,.91)$

(c) Nitric oxide diffusion rates are normally distributed in the population from which the sample was drawn.

(d) **Practical:** We are 95% confident the mean maximal nitric oxide diffusion rate for asthmatic schoolchildren is between 2.64 and 4.36 while for control subjects it is between .49 and .91. **Probabilistic:** approximately 95% of intervals constructed ina similar manner with samples of size 15 drawn from the populations of asthmatic and control schoolchildren will contain the respective population means.

(e) The practical.

(f)   Narrower because the t coefficient from which the interval is constructed is smaller.

(g)   Wider because the t coefficient from which the interval is constructed is larger.

6.3.5. $s_{\bar{x}} = 12/\sqrt{16} = 3$

90 % CI: $71.5 \pm 1.7530(3) = (66.2, 76.8)$

95 % CI: $71.5 \pm 2.1315(3) = (65.1, 77.9)$

99 % CI: $71.5 \pm 2.9467(3) = (62.7, 80.3)$

6.4.1. The samples constitute independent simple random samples from the two populations. The two populations of free fatty acid concentrations are normally distributed, and the two population variances are equal.

$$s_1 = 30\sqrt{18} = 127.2792, \quad s_2 = 62\sqrt{11} = 205.6307$$

$$s_p^2 = \frac{17(127.2792^2) + 10(205.6307^2)}{18 + 11 - 2} = 25860.7318, \quad s_p = \sqrt{25860.7318} = 160.8127$$

90% CI: $(299 - 744) \pm 1.7033\sqrt{\dfrac{25860.7318}{18} + \dfrac{25860.7318}{11}} = (-549.8, -340.2)$

95% CI: $(299 - 744) \pm 2.0518\sqrt{\dfrac{25860.7318}{18} + \dfrac{25860.7318}{11}} = (-571.3, -318.7)$

99% CI: $(299 - 744) \pm 2.7707\sqrt{\dfrac{25860.7318}{18} + \dfrac{25860.7318}{11}} = (-615.5, -274.5)$

6.4.3. The samples constitute independent simple random samples from the two populations. The two populations of pain scores are normally distributed, and the two population variances are equal.

$$s_1 = 5.5\sqrt{40} = 34.7851 \quad s_2 = 4.6\sqrt{57} = 34.7292$$

$$\sigma_{\bar{x}_1 - \bar{x}_2} = \sqrt{\frac{34.7851^2}{40} + \frac{34.7292^2}{57}} = 7.1701$$

90 % CI: $(36.4 - 30.5) \pm 1.645(7.1701) = (-5.89, 17.69)$

95 % CI: $(36.4 - 30.5) \pm 1.96(7.1701) = (-8.15, 19.95)$

99 % CI: $(36.4 - 30.5) \pm 2.58(7.1701) = (-12.60, 24.40)$

6.4.5. The samples constitute independent simple random samples from the two populations. The two populations of doses of methadone are normally distributed, and the two population variances are equal.

$$s_p^2 = \frac{8(156)^2 + 7(316)^2}{9 + 8 - 2} = 59578.6667, \ s_p = \sqrt{59578.6667} = 244.0874$$

90 % CI: $(541 - 269) \pm 1.7530 \sqrt{\dfrac{244.0874^2}{9} + \dfrac{244.0874^2}{8}} = (64.1, 479.9)$

95 % CI: $(541 - 269) \pm 2.1314 \sqrt{\dfrac{244.0874^2}{9} + \dfrac{244.0874^2}{8}} = (19.2, 524.8)$

99 % CI: $(541 - 269) \pm 2.9467 \sqrt{\dfrac{244.0874^2}{9} + \dfrac{244.0874^2}{8}} = (-77.5, 621.5)$

6.4.7. $s_p^2 = \dfrac{11(1.5)^2 + 11(2.0)^2}{11 + 11} = 3.125$

$s_{\bar{x}_1 - \bar{x}_2} = \sqrt{\dfrac{3.125}{12} + \dfrac{3.125}{12}} = .7217$

90 % CI: $(11.1 - 7.8) \pm 1.7171(.7217) = (2.1, 4.5)$

95 % CI: $(11.1 - 7.8) \pm 2.0739(.7217) = (1.8, 4.8)$

99 % CI: $(11.1 - 7.8) \pm 2.8188(.7217) = (1.3, 5.3)$

6.4.9. $\qquad s_{\overline{x}_1-\overline{x}_2} = \sqrt{\dfrac{4}{20}+\dfrac{100}{24}} = 2.089657$

90 % CI: $\qquad t'_{1-\alpha/2} = \dfrac{(4/20)(1.7291)+(100/24)(1.7139)}{(4/20)+(100/24)} = \dfrac{7.48707}{4.366667} = 1.7146$

$$(7-36)\pm 1.7146(2.089657) = (-32.58,-25.42)$$

95 % CI: $\qquad t'_{1-\alpha/2} = \dfrac{(4/20)(2.093)+(100/24)(2.0687)}{(4/20)+(100/24)} = \dfrac{9.038183}{4.366667} = 2.0698$

$$(7-36)\pm 2.0698(2.089657) = (-33.32,-24.67)$$

99 % CI: $\qquad t'_{1-\alpha/2} = \dfrac{(4/20)(2.8609)+(100/24)(2.8073)}{(4/20)+(100/24)} = \dfrac{12.269263}{4.366667} = 2.8098$

$$(7-36)\pm 2.8098(2.089657) = (-34.87,-23.13)$$

6.5.1. Point estimate: $\hat{p} = 63/472 = .1335$, $\qquad$ Reliability coefficient: 1.96

Standard error: $\sqrt{\dfrac{(.1335)(.8665)}{472}} = .0157$

CI: $.1335 \pm 1.96(.0157) = (.1027,.1643)$

Practical: We are 95% confident the true proportion of ventilator-associated pneumonia is between .1027 and .1643. **Probabilistic:** Approximately 95% of intervals constructed in a similar manner with samples of size 472 drawn from the populations of ventilated patients will contain the respective population proportion.

6.5.3. Point estimate: $\hat{p} = 75/136 = .5515$, $\qquad$ Reliability coefficient: 2.58

Standard error: $\sqrt{\dfrac{(.5515)(.4485)}{136}} = .0426$

CI: $.5515 \pm 2.58(.0426) = (.4415,.6615)$

6.6.1. Point estimates: $\hat{p}_1 = 114/637 = .1790$, $\hat{p}_2 = 57/510 = .1118$

Reliability coefficient: 1.96

Standard error: $\sqrt{\dfrac{(.1790)(.8210)}{637} + \dfrac{(.1118)(.8882)}{510}} = .0206$

CI: $(.1790 - .1118) \pm 1.96(.0206) = (.0268, .1076)$

Practical: We are 95% confident the true difference in proportions between the abused or neglected group and the control group is between .0268 and .1076. **Probabilistic:** Approximately 95% of intervals constructed in a similar manner with samples of size 637 and 510 drawn from the two populations will contain the difference in the respective population proportions.

6.6.3. Point estimates: $\hat{p}_1 = 16/49 = .3265$, $\hat{p}_2 = 12/51 = .2353$

Reliability coefficient: 1.96

Standard error: $\sqrt{\dfrac{(.3265)(.6735)}{49} + \dfrac{(.2353)(.7647)}{51}} = .0895$

CI: $(.3265 - .2353) \pm 1.96(.0895) = (-.0842, .2666)$

6.7.1. $n = \dfrac{(2.58)^2 (1)^2}{.5^2} = 26.6256 \approx 27$

$n = \dfrac{(1.96)^2 (1)^2}{.5^2} = 15.3664 \approx 16$

6.7.3. $n = \dfrac{(1.645)^2 (60)}{3^2} = 18.0402 \approx 19$

6.8.1. $n = \dfrac{(1.96)^2 (.20)(.80)}{(.03)^2} = 682.9511 \approx 683$

$n = \dfrac{(1.96)^2 (.5)(.5)}{(.03)^2} = 1067.1111 \approx 1068$

6.8.3. $n = \dfrac{(1.96)^2(.5)(.5)}{(.05)^2} = 384.16 \approx 385$

$n = \dfrac{(1.96)^2(.25)(.75)}{(.05)^2} = 288.12 \approx 289$

6.9.1. $s^2 = 13.3889, \; \chi_{.975} = 19.022, \; \chi_{.025} = 2.700$

$\dfrac{9(13.3889)}{19.023} < \sigma^2 < \dfrac{9(13.3889)}{2.700} \Rightarrow 6.334 < \sigma^2 < 44.630$

6.9.3. $\dfrac{19(1,000,000)}{30.144} < \sigma^2 < \dfrac{19(1,000,000)}{10.117}$

$630,307.86 < \sigma^2 < 1,878,027.08, \quad 793.92 < \sigma < 1370.41$

6.9.5. $\dfrac{24(2.25)}{39.364} < \sigma^2 < \dfrac{24(2.25)}{12.401}$

$1.37 < \sigma^2 < 4.35, \quad 1.17 < \sigma < 2.09$

6.9.7. $s^2 = 295.6421, \; \dfrac{19(295.6421)}{32.852} < \sigma^2 < \dfrac{19(295.6421)}{8.907}$

$170.0985 < \sigma^2 < 630.6500$

6.10.1. $s^2_{Incomplete} = 10.9652, \; s^2_{Complete} = 5.5824, \; n_{Incomplete} = 5, \; n_{Complete} = 11$

$\dfrac{s^2_{Incomplete}}{s^2_{Complete}} = \dfrac{10.9652}{5.5824} = 1.9642$

$\dfrac{1.9642}{4.47} < \dfrac{\sigma^2_{Incomplete}}{\sigma^2_{Complete}} < \dfrac{1.9642}{.1131} \Rightarrow .44 < \dfrac{\sigma^2_{Incomplete}}{\sigma^2_{Complete}} < 17.37$

6.10.3. $\dfrac{12/10}{2.46} < \dfrac{\sigma^2_1}{\sigma^2_2} < \dfrac{12/10}{1/2.46} \Rightarrow .49 < \dfrac{\sigma^2_1}{\sigma^2_2} < 2.95$

6.10.5. $\dfrac{35,000/20,000}{1.94} < \dfrac{\sigma^2_1}{\sigma^2_2} < \dfrac{35,000/20,000}{1/2.01} \Rightarrow .90 < \dfrac{\sigma^2_1}{\sigma^2_2} < 3.52$

6.10.7. $s_N^2 = 4.066625,$ $s_U^2 = 65.042333,$ $\dfrac{s_U^2}{s_N^2} = \dfrac{65.042333}{4.066625} = 15.99418$

$$\dfrac{15.99418}{3.12} < \dfrac{\sigma_1^2}{\sigma_2^2} < \dfrac{15.99418}{1/3.77} \Rightarrow 5.13 < \dfrac{\sigma_1^2}{\sigma_2^2} < 60.30$$

Chapter 6 Review Exercises

13. $\bar{x} = 79.87, s^2 = 28.1238, s = 5.3;\ 79.87 \pm 2.1448\left(5.30/\sqrt{15}\right) = (76.93, 82.81)$

15. $\hat{p} = 21/70 = .30,\ .30 \pm 1.96\sqrt{(.3)(.7)/70} = (.19, .41)$

17. $\hat{p}_1 = 44/220 = .20,\ \hat{p}_2 = 150/280 = .54$

$$(.54 - .20) \pm 1.96\sqrt{\dfrac{(.54)(.46)}{280} + \dfrac{(.20)(.80)}{220}} = (.26, .42)$$

19. $\hat{p} = 180/200 = .90,\ .90 \pm 1.645\sqrt{\dfrac{(.9)(.1)}{200}} = (.87, .93)$

21. $\bar{x} = 19.23,\ s^2 = 20.2268;\ 19.23 \pm 2.2622\sqrt{20.2268)/10} = (16.01, 22.45)$

23. $\bar{x}_A = 6.125,\ s_A^2 = 15.8420,\ \bar{x}_B = 5.806,\ s_B^2 = 5.9980$

$$s_p^2 = \dfrac{11(15.8420) + 15(5.9980)}{11 + 15} = 10.1628$$

$$(6.125 - 5.8420) \pm 2.0555\sqrt{\dfrac{10.1628}{12} + \dfrac{10.1628}{16}} = (-2.18, 2.82)$$

25. $435 \pm 1.96\dfrac{215}{\sqrt{34}} = (362.73, 507.27)$

27. $\hat{p} = 23/39 = .5897,\ .5897 \pm 1.96\sqrt{\dfrac{(.5897)(.4103)}{39}} = (.4353, .7441)$

29. $s_{CP} = (.0582)\sqrt{10} = .1840, \ s_C = (.1641)\sqrt{10} = .5189$

Assume equal variances for the two groups, $s_p^2 = \dfrac{9(.1840)^2 + 9(.5189)^2}{18} = .1516$

$(.220 - .334) \pm 1.7341\sqrt{\dfrac{.1516}{10} + \dfrac{.1516}{10}} = (-.416, .188)$

31.   Level of confidence decreases. The interval would have no width. The level of confidence would be zero.

33.   Since the sample size is 32, the reliability coefficient should be z.
The precision of the estimate equals the margin of error, which is 8.1

35.   All drivers aged 55 and older. Drivers 55 and older participating in the vision study.

37. $\bar{x} = .3197, \ s = .2486, \ n = 216$

$.3197 \pm 1.96\dfrac{.2486}{\sqrt{216}} = (.2865, .3529)$

We use z since $n > 30$.

Chapter 7

7.2.1. $H_0 : \mu \geq 75,\ H_A : \mu < 75,\ z = \dfrac{70.7 - 75}{\left(14.6/\sqrt{76}\right)} = -2.57$

Reject H_0 since $-2.57 < -2.33, p = .0051 < .01$

7.2.3. $H_0 : \mu \leq 9,\ H_A : \mu > 9,\ t = \dfrac{10.3 - 9}{\left(7.3/\sqrt{18}\right)} = .76$

Fail to reject H_0 since $.76 < 1.333, p > .10$

7.2.5. $H_0 : \mu \geq 30,\ H_A : \mu < 30,\ z = \dfrac{21 - 30}{\left(11/\sqrt{49}\right)} = -5.73$

Yes, Reject H_0 since $z = -5.73 < -1.645, p < .0001$

7.2.7. $H_0 : \mu \geq 80,\ H_A : \mu < 80,\ t = \dfrac{77 - 80}{\left(10/\sqrt{25}\right)} = -1.50$

Fail to reject H_0 since $t = -1.50 > -1.7109, .05 < p < .10$

7.2.9. $H_0 : \mu \leq 25;\ H_A : \mu > 25;\ z = \dfrac{27 - 25}{\left(6.5/\sqrt{100}\right)} = 3.08$

Reject H_0 since $z = 3.08 > 1.645, p = .0010$

7.2.11. $H_0 : \mu \leq 10,\ H_A : \mu > 10,\ z = \dfrac{13 - 10}{\left(3/\sqrt{16}\right)} = 4.0$

Reject H_0 since $z = 4.0 > 1.645, p < .0001$

7.2.13. $H_0 : \mu = 110,\ H_A : \mu \neq 110,\ t = \dfrac{111.60 - 110}{\left(56.303/\sqrt{20}\right)} = .1271$

Fail to Reject H_0 since $t = .1271 < 2.8609, p > .1(2) = .2$

7.2.15. $H_0 : \mu \geq 30, \; H_A : \mu < 30, \; z = \dfrac{19.46 - 30}{17.8171/\sqrt{50}} = -4.18$

Reject H_0 since $z = -4.18 > 1.645, p < .0001$

7.2.17. $H_0 : \mu = 100, \; H_A : \mu \neq 100, \; z = \dfrac{105 - 100}{15/\sqrt{25}} = 1.67$

Fail to reject H_0 since $z = 1.67 < 1.96, p = 2(.0475) = .095$

7.2.19. $H_0 : \mu \leq 70, \; H_A : \mu > 70, \; z = \dfrac{63 - 70}{7/\sqrt{16}} = -4.00$

Reject H_0 since $z = -4.00 < -2.33, p < .0001$

7.3.1. $H_0 : \mu_{MS} \geq \mu_R, \; H_A : \mu_{MS} < \mu_R, \; s_p^2 = \dfrac{39(1.27^2) + 23(2.64)^2}{62} = 3.6001$

$$t = \dfrac{(22.41 - 27.75)}{\sqrt{\dfrac{3.6001}{40} + \dfrac{3.6001}{24}}} = -10.9001$$

Reject H_0 since $-10.9001 < -2.388, p < .005$

7.3.3. $H_0 : \mu_{NOSAS} = \mu_{OSAS}, \; H_A : \mu_{NOSAS} \neq \mu_{OSAS}$

$$s_p^2 = \dfrac{36(5.5890^2) + 25(6.9568)^2}{61} = 38.2698; \; t = \dfrac{(95.854 - 111.060)}{\sqrt{\dfrac{38.2698}{37} + \dfrac{38.2698}{26}}} = -9.61$$

Reject H_0 since $-9.61 < -2.6591, p < .005(2)$

7.3.5. $H_0 : \mu_I = \mu_C, \; H_A : \mu_I \neq \mu_C, \; z = \dfrac{(12.341 - 5.317)}{\sqrt{\dfrac{10.5726^2}{41} + \dfrac{8.0450^2}{41}}} = 3.39$

Reject H_0 since $z = 3.39 > 1.96, p = .0003$

7.3.7. $H_0 : \mu_1 = \mu_2, \ H_A : \mu_1 \neq \mu_2$

$$s_p^2 = \frac{9(65)^2 + 11(80)^2}{9 + 11} = 5421.25, \ t = \frac{435 - 645}{\sqrt{\dfrac{5421.25}{10} + \dfrac{5421.35}{12}}} = -6.66$$

Reject H_0 since $-6.66 < -2.0860, p < 2(.005) = .010$

7.3.9. $H_0 : \mu_1 = \mu_2, \ H_A : \mu_1 \neq \mu_2, \ z = \dfrac{(8.5 - 4.8)}{\sqrt{\dfrac{5.5^2}{35} + \dfrac{3.6^2}{40}}} = 3.39$

Reject H_0 since $z = 3.39 > 1.96, p = .0003(2) = .0006$

7.3.11. $\bar{x}_A = 10.28, \ s_A = .5978, \ \bar{x}_B = 11.08, \ s_B = .4590$

$$H_0 : \mu_A = \mu_B; \ H_A : \mu_A \neq \mu_B$$

$$s_p^2 = \frac{9(.5978^2) + 9(.4590)^2}{18} = .2840, \ t = \frac{(10.28 - 11.08)}{\sqrt{\dfrac{.284}{10} + \dfrac{.284}{10}}} = -3.3567$$

Reject H_0 since $t = -3.3567 < -2.1009, p < .005(2) = .010$

7.4.1. $d_i = $ Pre-Post, $H_0 : \mu_d \leq 0, \ H_A : \mu_d > 0$

$$\bar{d} = 1.60, \ s = 1.9567, \ t = \frac{1.60}{(1.9567/\sqrt{15})} = 3.17$$

Reject H_0 since $3.17 > 2.624, p < .005$

7.4.3. $d_i = $ Methdone - Placebo $H_0 : \mu_d \geq 0, \ H_A : \mu_d < 0$

$$\bar{d} = -9.618, \ s = 10.1096, \ t = \frac{-9.618}{(10.1096/\sqrt{11})} = -3.1553$$

Reject H_0 since $-3.1553 < -1.8125, .005 < p < .01$

7.4.5. $d_i =$ Base - Follow-up $H_0 : \mu_d = 0,\ H_A : \mu_d \neq 0$

$$\overline{d} = -144.4286,\ s = 85.6774,\ t = \frac{-144.4286}{(85.6774/\sqrt{7})} = -4.4600$$

Reject H_0 since -4.4600 < -2.4469, $p < .005(2) = .0100$

7.5.1. $H_0 : p \geq .35,\ H_A : p < .35;\ \hat{p} = 90/295 = .3051$

$$z = \frac{.3051 - .35}{\sqrt{\dfrac{(.35)(.65)}{295}}} = -1.62 \quad \text{Fail to reject } H_0 \text{ since } -1.62 > -1.645,\ p = .0526$$

7.5.3. $H_0 : p \geq .20,\ H_A : p < .20;\ \hat{p} = 5/50 = .10$

$$z = \frac{.10 - .20}{\sqrt{\dfrac{(.20)(.80)}{50}}} = -1.77 \quad \text{Reject } H_0 \text{ since } -1.77 < -1.645,\ p = .0384$$

7.5.5. $H_0 : p \geq .15,\ H_A : p < .15;\ \hat{p} = 25/250 = .10$

$$z = \frac{.10 - .15}{\sqrt{\dfrac{(.15)(.85)}{250}}} = -2.21 \quad \text{Reject } H_0 \text{ since } z = -2.21 < -1.645,\ p = .0136$$

7.6.1. $\hat{p}_C = 72/1222 = .0589,\ \hat{p}_F = 30/282 = .1064,\ \overline{p} = \dfrac{72+30}{1222+282} = .0678$

$$H_0 : p_C = p_F,\ H_A : p_C \neq p_F,\ z = \frac{(.0589 - .1064)}{\sqrt{\dfrac{.0678(.9322)}{1222} + \dfrac{.0678(.9322)}{282}}} = -2.86$$

Reject H_0 since -2.86 < - 2.58, $p = .0042$

7.6.3. $\hat{p}_{Hemo} = 249/529 = .4707,\ \hat{p}_{Peri} = 134/326 = .4110,\ \overline{p} = \dfrac{249+134}{529+326} = .4480$

$$H_0 : p_{Hemo} = p_{Peri},\ H_A : p_{Hemo} \neq p_{Peri},\ z = \frac{(.4707 - .4110)}{\sqrt{\dfrac{.4480(.5520)}{529} + \dfrac{.4480(.5520)}{326}}} = 1.70$$

Fail to reject H_0 since 1.70 < 1.96, $p = .0314(2) = .0628$

7.7.1. $H_0 : \sigma^2 = 20,\ H_A : \sigma^2 \neq 20,\ s^2 = 25.9044$

$$\chi^2 = \frac{16(25.9044)}{20} = 20.723$$

Do not reject H_0 since $5.142 < 20.723 < 34.267,\ p > .01$ (two-sided test).

7.7.3. $H_0 : \sigma^2 = 1,\ H_A : \sigma^2 \neq 1,\ s^2 = .75$

$$\chi^2 = \frac{9(.75)}{1} = 6.75$$

Do not reject H_0 since $2.700 < 6.75 < 19.023,\ p > .05$ (two-sided test)

7.7.5. $H_0 : \sigma^2 \leq 25,\ H_A : \sigma^2 > 25,\ s^2 = 30$

$$\chi^2 = \frac{24(30)}{25} = 28.8$$

Do not reject H_0 since $28.8 < 36.415,\ p > .10$

7.7.7. $H_0 : \sigma^2 \leq .05,\ H_A : \sigma^2 > .05,\ s^2 = .0787$

$$\chi^2 = \frac{14(.0787)}{.05} = 22.036$$

Do not reject H_0 since $22.036 < 23.685,\ .05 < p < .10$

7.8.1. $H_0 : \sigma_D^2 \leq \sigma_C^2 \quad H_A : \sigma_D^2 > \sigma_C^2,\ s_D^2 = 3.1^2 = 9.61,\ s_C^2 = 2.8^2 = 7.84,\ n_D = 30,\ n_C = 45$

$$\text{V.R.} = \frac{9.61}{7.84} = 1.226$$

Fail to reject H_0 since V.R. $= 1.226 < 1.74,\ p > .10$

7.8.3. $H_0 : \sigma_F^2 \leq \sigma_M^2$ $H_A : \sigma_F^2 > \sigma_M^2$, $s_F^2 = 275$, $s_M^2 = 150$, $n_F = 21$, $n_M = 16$

$$\text{V.R.} = \frac{275}{150} = 1.83$$

Fail to reject H_0 since V.R. = $1.83 < 2.33$, $p > .10$

7.8.5. $H_0 : \sigma_1^2 = \sigma_2^2$ $H_A : \sigma_1^2 \neq \sigma_2^2$, $s_1^2 = 64$, $s_2^2 = 16$, $n_E = 13$, $n_{NE} = 13$

$$\text{V.R.} = \frac{64}{16} = 4.0$$

Reject H_0 since V.R. = $4 > 3.28$, $.01(2) < p < .025(2)$, $.02 < p < .05$

7.8.7. $H_0 : \sigma_A^2 \leq \sigma_B^2$ $H_A : \sigma_A^2 > \sigma_B^2$, $s_A^2 = 852.9333$, $s_B^2 = 398.2424$, $n_A = 10$, $n_B = 12$

$$\text{V.R.} = \frac{852.3333}{398.2424} = 2.14$$

Fail to reject H_0 since V.R. = $2.14 < 2.90$, $p > .10$

7.9.1.

Alternative Value of μ	β	Value of Power Function $1-\beta$
516	0.9500	0.0500
521	0.8461	0.1539
528	0.5596	0.4404
533	0.3156	0.6844
539	0.1093	0.8907
544	0.0314	0.9686
547	0.0129	0.9871

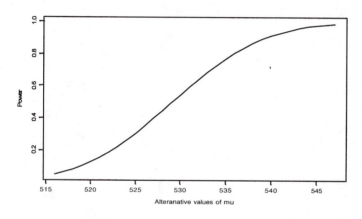

7.9.3.

Alternative Value of μ	β	Value of Power Function $1-\beta$
4.25	0.9900	0.0100
4.50	0.8599	0.1401
4.75	0.4325	0.5675
5.00	0.0778	0.9222
5.25	0.0038	0.9962

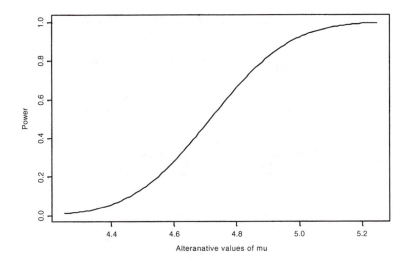

7.10.1. $n = \left[\dfrac{(1.645 + 1.28)(32)}{516 - 520} \right]^2 = 547.56 \approx 548$

$$C = 516 + 1.645\left(\frac{32}{\sqrt{548}}\right) = 518.25, \ \ C = 520 - 1.28\left(\frac{32}{\sqrt{548}}\right) = 518.25$$

Select a sample of size 548 and compute $\overline{x}$. If $\overline{x} \geq$ 518.25, reject H_0.
If $\overline{x}$ < 518.25, do not reject H_0.

7.10.3. $n = \left[\dfrac{(2.33 + 1.88)(1.8)}{4.25 - 5.00} \right]^2 = 102.09 \approx 103$

$$C = 4.25 + 2.33\left(\frac{1.8}{\sqrt{103}}\right) = 4.66, \ \ C = 5.00 - 1.88\left(\frac{1.8}{\sqrt{103}}\right) = 4.67$$

Select a sample of size 103 and compute $\overline{x}$. If $\overline{x} \geq$ 4.66, reject H_0.
If $\overline{x}$ < 4.66, do not reject H_0.

Chapter 7 Review Exercises

19. $H_0 : \mu_d \leq 0, \; H_A : \mu_d > 0, \; d_i = \text{Before - After}, \bar{d} = 79.43, \; s_d = 27.8561$

$$z = \frac{79.43}{27.8564/\sqrt{107}} = 29.50 \quad \text{Reject } H_0 \text{ since } 29.49 > 2.33, p < .0001$$

21. $H_0 : p_V = p_S, \; H_A : p_V \neq p_S, \; \hat{p}_V = 115/122 = .9426, \; \hat{p}_2 = 87/98 = .8878$

$$\bar{p} = \frac{(115+87)}{(122+98)} = .9182, \quad z = \frac{(.9426 - .8878)}{\sqrt{\frac{(.9182)(.0818)}{122} + \frac{(.9182)(.0818)}{98}}} = 1.47$$

Fail to reject the null since $z = 1.47 < 1.96, \; p = .1416$

23. $H_0 : \mu_C = \mu_H, \; H_A : \mu_C \neq \mu_H, s_C = .07\sqrt{208} = 1.0096, \; s_H = .05\sqrt{19} = .2179$

$$z = \frac{(1.81 - .71)}{\sqrt{\frac{1.0096^2}{208} + \frac{.2179^2}{19}}} = 12.79$$

Reject H_0 since $12.79 > 2.58, p < .0001$

25. $H_0 : p \leq .25, \; H_A : p > .25, \; \hat{p} = 27/90 = .30, \; z = \frac{(.30 - .25)}{\sqrt{\frac{(.25)(.75)}{90}}} = 1.10$

Fail to reject H_0 since $1.10 < 1.645, p = .1357$

27. $H_0 : \mu \leq 40, \; H_A : \mu > 40, \; t = \frac{(45 - 40)}{\left(5/\sqrt{15}\right)} = 3.873$

Reject H_0 since $3.873 > 1.7613, p < .005$

29. $H_0 : \mu_d \leq 0, \; H_A : \mu_d > 0, \; d_i = \text{Nonsmoking - Smoking}, \bar{d} = 11.49, \; s_d = 16.02$

$$t = \frac{11.49}{\left(16.02/\sqrt{12}\right)} = 2.485, \quad \text{Reject } H_0 \text{ since } 2.486 > 1.7959, .025 > p > .01$$

31. $H_0 : \mu \geq 2000, \ H_A : \mu < 2000, \ t = \dfrac{(1600 - 2000)}{\left(700/\sqrt{16}\right)} = -2.286$

Reject H_0 since $-2.286 < -1.7530, \ .01 < p < .025$

41.　One-Sample T: Diff

Test of mu = 0 vs not = 0

Variable	N	Mean	StDev	SE Mean	95% CI	T	P
Diff	11	666.364	311.790	94.008	(456.900, 875.827)	7.09	0.000

43.　One-Sample T: Diff

Test of mu = 0 vs not = 0

Variable	N	Mean	StDev	SE Mean	95% CI	T	P
Diff	31	0.510323	0.779489	0.140000	(0.224404, 0.796242)	3.65	0.001

45. Paired T-Test and CI: LEGB, LEGA

Paired T for LEGB - LEGA

	N	Mean	StDev	SE Mean
LEGB	15	111.667	27.430	7.082
LEGA	15	156.000	34.132	8.813
Difference	15	-44.3333	21.8654	5.6456

95% CI for mean difference: (-56.4420, -32.2247)
T-Test of mean difference = 0 (vs not = 0): T-Value = -7.85　P-Value = 0.000

Paired T-Test and CI: HIPFB, HIPFA

Paired T for HIPFB - HIPFA

	N	Mean	StDev	SE Mean
HIPFB	15	8.2667	2.2509	0.5812
HIPFA	15	13.0000	4.0532	1.0465
Difference	15	-4.73333	2.98727	0.77131

95% CI for mean difference: (-6.38763, -3.07904)
T-Test of mean difference = 0 (vs not = 0): T-Value = -6.14　P-Value = 0.000

Paired T-Test and CI: HIPEB, HIPEA

```
Paired T for HIPEB - HIPEA

              N      Mean    StDev   SE Mean
HIPEB        15   11.2000   2.7826   0.7185
HIPEA        15   19.3333   6.1023   1.5756
Difference   15  -8.13333  3.79599  0.98012


95% CI for mean difference: (-10.23548, -6.03119)
T-Test of mean difference = 0 (vs not = 0): T-Value = -8.30  P-Value = 0.000
```

Paired T-Test and CI: ARMABDB, ARMABDA

```
Paired T for ARMABDB - ARMABDA

              N      Mean    StDev   SE Mean
ARMABDB      15    7.3333   2.3805   0.6146
ARMABDA      15   12.8000   3.8023   0.9817
Difference   15  -5.46667  3.15926  0.81572


95% CI for mean difference: (-7.21621, -3.71712)
T-Test of mean difference = 0 (vs not = 0): T-Value = -6.70  P-Value = 0.000
```

Paired T-Test and CI: ARMADDB, ARMADDA

```
Paired T for ARMADDB - ARMADDA

              N      Mean    StDev   SE Mean
ARMADDB      15    8.8667   2.8251   0.7294
ARMADDA      15   15.0000   3.9461   1.0189
Difference   15  -6.13333  2.77403  0.71625


95% CI for mean difference: (-7.66954, -4.59713)
T-Test of mean difference = 0 (vs not = 0): T-Value = -8.56  P-Value = 0.000
```

47. Paired T-Test and CI: PRE, POST

```
Paired T for PRE - POST

              N      Mean    StDev   SE Mean
PRE          66   392.439  125.950   15.503
POST         66   343.242  105.432   12.978
Difference   66   49.1970  92.1966  11.3486


95% CI for mean difference: (26.5322, 71.8617)
T-Test of mean difference = 0 (vs not = 0): T-Value = 4.34  P-Value = 0.000
```

49. Two-Sample T-Test and CI: NOASTH, ASTH

```
Two-sample T for NOASTH vs ASTH

          N   Mean   StDev  SE Mean
NOASTH   22   56.1    43.0      9.2
ASTH     22  108.0    60.0       13


Difference = mu (NOASTH) - mu (ASTH)
Estimate for difference:  -51.8977
95% CI for difference:  (-83.6549, -20.1405)
T-Test of difference = 0 (vs not =): T-Value = -3.30  P-Value = 0.002  DF = 42
Both use Pooled StDev = 52.1915
```

51. Two-Sample T-Test and CI: ACID, GROUP

```
Two-sample T for ACID

GROUP      N   Mean   StDev  SE Mean
1.000000   5   15.9    10.1      4.5
2.000000  17   2.48    4.45      1.1


Difference = mu (1.000000) - mu (2.000000)
Estimate for difference:  13.4435
95% CI for difference:  (0.4957, 26.3914)
T-Test of difference = 0 (vs not =): T-Value = 2.88  P-Value = 0.045  DF = 4
```

53. Two-Sample T-Test and CI: Scores, Group

```
Two-sample T for Scores

Group      N   Mean   StDev  SE Mean
1.000000  27   2.26    4.11     0.79
2.000000  28   2.64    5.46      1.0


Difference = mu (1.000000) - mu (2.000000)
Estimate for difference:  -0.383598
95% CI for difference:  (-2.994477, 2.227281)
T-Test of difference = 0 (vs not =): T-Value = -0.30  P-Value = 0.769  DF = 50
```

55. Two-Sample T-Test and CI: Scores, Group

```
Two-sample T for Scores

Group      N   Mean   StDev  SE Mean
1.000000  24   18.8    12.4      2.5
2.000000  26   5.62    5.49      1.1


Difference = mu (1.000000) - mu (2.000000)
Estimate for difference:  13.1763
95% CI for difference:  (7.5541, 18.7985)
T-Test of difference = 0 (vs not =): T-Value = 4.78  P-Value = 0.000  DF = 31
```

Chapter 8

Answers for 8.2.1-8.2.7 obtained by SAS®

8.2.1.   The MEANS Procedure

Analysis Variable : EMT

ANGLE	N Obs	N	Mean	Std Dev	Minimum	Maximum
30	69	69	0.6877391	0.7975196	-1.1640000	2.7330000
60	33	33	0.2401515	0.9769852	-1.1890000	2.7270000
90	194	194	0.8787990	1.1203785	-2.8620000	2.7620000
120	33	33	0.2441818	0.9867145	-1.1800000	2.7630000

Dependent Variable: EMT

Source	DF	Sum of Squares	Mean Square	F Value	Pr > F
Model	3	20.0070713	6.6690238	6.24	0.0004
Error	325	347.2127836	1.0683470		
Corrected Total	328	367.2198549			

$$HSD_{30,60}* = q_{.05,4,325}\sqrt{\frac{1.608347}{2}\left(\frac{1}{69}+\frac{1}{33}\right)} = 3.65207*.1897988 = .6931$$

Since $.6877 - .2402 = .4475 < .6931, \overline{x}_{30} - \overline{x}_{60}$ is not significant.

$$HSD_{30,90}* = q_{.05,4,325}\sqrt{\frac{1.608347}{2}\left(\frac{1}{69}+\frac{1}{194}\right)} = 3.65207*.1256878 = .4591$$

Since $\left|.6877 - .8788\right| = .1911 < .6931, \overline{x}_{30} - \overline{x}_{90}$ is not significant.

$$HSD_{30,120}* = q_{.05,4,325}\sqrt{\frac{1.608347}{2}\left(\frac{1}{69}+\frac{1}{33}\right)} = 3.65207*.1897988 = .6931$$

Since $.6877 - .2442 = .4435 < .6931, \overline{x}_{30} - \overline{x}_{60}$ is not significant.

$$HSD_{60,90}* = q_{.05,4,325}\sqrt{\frac{1.608347}{2}\left(\frac{1}{33}+\frac{1}{194}\right)} = 3.65207*.16886 = .6167$$

Since $\left|.2402 - .8788\right| = .6386 > .6137, \overline{x}_{60} - \overline{x}_{90}$ is significant.

$$HSD_{60,120}* = q_{.05,4,325}\sqrt{\frac{1.608347}{2}\left(\frac{1}{33}+\frac{1}{33}\right)} = 3.65207*.22077 = .8063$$

Since $\left|.2402 - .2442\right| = .0004 < .8063, \overline{x}_{60} - \overline{x}_{120}$ is not significant.

$$HSD_{90,120}* = q_{.05,4,325}\sqrt{\frac{1.608347}{2}\left(\frac{1}{194}+\frac{1}{33}\right)} = 3.65207*.16886 = .6167$$

Since $\left|.8788 - .2442\right| = .6346 > .6167, \overline{x}_{90} - \overline{x}_{120}$ is significant.

Alpha	0.05
Error Degrees of Freedom	325
Error Mean Square	1.068347
Critical Value of Studentized Range	3.65207

Comparisons significant at the 0.05 level are indicated by ***.

group Comparison		Difference Between Means	Simultaneous 95% Confidence Limits		
90	- 30	0.1911	-0.1831	0.5652	
90	-120	0.6346	0.1320	1.1372	***
90	- 60	0.6386	0.1360	1.1413	***
30	- 90	-0.1911	-0.5652	0.1831	
30	-120	0.4436	-0.1214	1.0085	
30	- 60	0.4476	-0.1173	1.0125	
120	- 90	-0.6346	-1.1372	-0.1320	***
120	- 30	-0.4436	-1.0085	0.1214	
120	- 60	0.0040	-0.6531	0.6611	
60	- 90	-0.6386	-1.1413	-0.1360	***
60	- 30	-0.4476	-1.0125	0.1173	
60	-120	-0.0040	-0.6611	0.6531	

8.2.3.

Analysis Variable : calcium

Group	N Obs	N	Mean	Std Dev	Minimum	Maximum
A	22	22	1448.36	629.1259655	222.0000000	2670.00
B	14	14	992.6428571	627.2629932	136.0000000	2408.00
C	29	29	873.8275862	304.7434599	239.0000000	1692.00
D	48	48	851.7291667	385.9066550	42.0000000	1781.00

Dependent Variable: calcium

Source	DF	Sum of Squares	Mean Square	F Value	Pr > F
Model	3	5931208.04	1977069.35	9.36	<.0001
Error	109	23026499.92	211252.29		
Corrected Total	112	28957707.96			

Pair	A vs B	A vs. C	A vs. D	B vs. C	B vs. D	C vs. D
HSD*	409.9861	339.0533	308.7524	390.2694	364.2541	282.0454

Alpha	0.05
Error Degrees of Freedom	109
Error Mean Square	211252.3
Critical Value of Studentized Range	3.68984

Comparisons significant at the 0.05 level are indicated by ***.

Group Comparison		Difference Between Means	Simultaneous 95% Confidence Limits		
A	- B	455.72	45.73	865.71	***
A	- C	574.54	235.48	913.59	***
A	- D	596.63	287.88	905.39	***
B	- A	-455.72	-865.71	-45.73	***
B	- C	118.82	-271.45	509.09	
B	- D	140.91	-223.34	505.17	
C	- A	-574.54	-913.59	-235.48	***
C	- B	-118.82	-509.09	271.45	
C	- D	22.10	-259.95	304.14	
D	- A	-596.63	-905.39	-287.88	***
D	- B	-140.91	-505.17	223.34	
D	- C	-22.10	-304.14	259.95	

8.2.5. Analysis Variable : force

Group	N Obs	N	Mean	Std Dev	Minimum	Maximum
E	10	10	70.0700000	16.4435769	51.9000000	96.0000000
MA	9	9	100.0444444	19.1217227	72.8000000	126.5000000
Y	10	10	118.2000000	35.2976864	74.0000000	193.6000000

Dependent Variable: force

Source	DF	Sum of Squares	Mean Square	F Value	Pr > F
Model	2	11799.23885	5899.61942	9.26	0.0009
Error	26	16571.98322	637.38397		
Corrected Total	28	28371.22207			

Pair	E vs. MA	E vs. Y	MA vs. Y
HSD*	28.8246	28.0558	28.8246

Alpha	0.05
Error Degrees of Freedom	26
Error Mean Square	637.384
Critical Value of Studentized Range	3.51417

Comparisons significant at the 0.05 level are indicated by ***.

Group Comparison			Difference Between Means	Simultaneous 95% Confidence Limits		
Y	-	MA	18.16	-10.67	46.98	
Y	-	E	48.13	20.07	76.19	***
MA	-	Y	-18.16	-46.98	10.67	
MA	-	E	29.97	1.15	58.80	***
E	-	Y	-48.13	-76.19	-20.07	***
E	-	MA	-29.97	-58.80	-1.15	***

8.2.7.
The MEANS Procedure

Analysis Variable : plate

Group	N Obs	N	Mean	Std Dev	Minimum	Maximum
0	67	67	2.1829851	0.3971375	0.8500000	2.8400000
1	30	30	2.0813333	0.4383884	0.7900000	2.7400000
2	54	54	2.0048148	0.4635171	0.7000000	2.8100000
3	27	27	1.8285185	0.3706927	1.0000000	2.4900000

Dependent Variable: plate

Source	DF	Sum of Squares	Mean Square	F Value	Pr > F
Model	3	2.63757326	0.87919109	4.94	0.0026
Error	174	30.94243854	0.17783011		
Corrected Total	177	33.58001180			

Pair	0 vs. 1	0 vs. 2	0 vs. 3	1 vs. 2	1 vs. 3	2 vs. 3
HSD*	.2403	.2000	.2494	.2491	.2902	.2578

Alpha	0.05
Error Degrees of Freedom	174
Error Mean Square	0.17783
Critical Value of Studentized Range	3.66853

Comparisons significant at the 0.05 level are indicated by ***.

Group Comparison		Difference Between Means	Simultaneous 95% Confidence Limits		
0	- 1	0.10165	-0.13866	0.34196	
0	- 2	0.17817	-0.02188	0.37822	
0	- 3	0.35447	0.10511	0.60383	***
1	- 0	-0.10165	-0.34196	0.13866	
1	- 2	0.07652	-0.17257	0.32561	
1	- 3	0.25281	-0.03737	0.54300	
2	- 0	-0.17817	-0.37822	0.02188	
2	- 1	-0.07652	-0.32561	0.17257	
2	- 3	0.17630	-0.08154	0.43413	
3	- 0	-0.35447	-0.60383	-0.10511	***
3	- 1	-0.25281	-0.54300	0.03737	
3	- 2	-0.17630	-0.43413	0.08154	

8.2.9. Treatment variable: HIV/PI treatment

Response variable: Percent body fat in the trunk

Extraneous variables: diet, exercise, viral load count

Treatments: HIV+, PI, and lipodystrophy; HIV+, PI, but no lipodystrophy; HIV+, no PI, No lipodystrophy; HIV-, no PI, and no lipdystrophy

The subjects are the patients enrolled in the study.

The HIV- men acted as a "control" group that would not regularly have lipodystrophy

Source	SS	df	MS	VR
Treatment		3		
Error		70		
Total		73		

8.3.1. Results for: EXR_C08_S03_01.mtw

Two-way ANOVA: score versus subject, type

```
Source    DF       SS       MS      F      P
subject   23   481.13   20.918   2.49  0.002
type       3   498.38  166.125  19.79  0.000
Error     69   579.13    8.393
Total     95  1558.63

S = 2.897   R-Sq = 62.84%   R-Sq(adj) = 48.84%
```

8.3.3. Results for: EXR_C08_S03_03.mtw

Two-way ANOVA: SCORE versus METHOD, MOTIV

```
Source    DF      SS       MS      F      P
METHOD     4   632.8  158.200  30.23  0.000
MOTIV      3   471.2  157.067  30.01  0.000
Error     12    62.8    5.233
Total     19  1166.8

S = 2.288   R-Sq = 94.62%   R-Sq(adj) = 91.48%
```

8.3.5. Results for: EXR_C08_S03_05.mtw

Two-way ANOVA: STRESS versus SUBJ, TREAT

```
Source    DF       SS       MS      F      P
SUBJ       3  260.667  86.8889  14.15  0.004
TREAT      2   90.500  45.2500   7.37  0.024
Error      6   36.833   6.1389
Total     11  388.000

S = 2.478   R-Sq = 90.51%   R-Sq(adj) = 82.60%
```

8.3.7.

Source	df
Blocks	5
Treatments	56
Error	30
Total	41

8.4.1. Results for: EXR_C08_S04_01.mtw

Two-way ANOVA: outcome versus subj, time

```
Source    DF       SS       MS      F      P
subj       9   64.225   7.1361   5.43  0.000
time       3  192.275  64.0917  48.78  0.000
Error     27   35.475   1.3139
Total     39  291.975

S = 1.146   R-Sq = 87.85%   R-Sq(adj) = 82.45%
```

8.4.3. Results for: EXR_C08_S04_03.mtw

Two-way ANOVA: SEINTAKE versus SUBJ, YEAR

```
Source  DF       SS       MS      F      P
SUBJ    15   3451.1   230.07   1.27  0.277
YEAR     2   5940.4  2970.19  16.45  0.000
Error   30   5415.7   180.52
Total   47  14807.2

S = 13.44   R-Sq = 63.43%   R-Sq(adj) = 42.70%
```

8.4.5.

Source	df
Subject	9
Time	2
Error	18
Total	29

8.5.1. Results for: EXR_C08_S05_01.mtw

Two-way ANOVA: Percent versus Treat, Dose

```
Source        DF       SS       MS      F      P
Treat          1   2021.8   2021.8   6.18  0.023
Dose           2  48765.6  24382.8  74.59  0.000
Interaction    2    583.7    291.9   0.89  0.427
Error         18   5884.1    326.9
Total         23  57255.2

S = 18.08   R-Sq = 89.72%   R-Sq(adj) = 86.87%
```

Two-way ANOVA: Percent versus Treat, Dose

```
Source  DF       SS       MS      F      P
Treat    1   2021.8   2021.8   6.25  0.021
Dose     2  48765.6  24382.8  75.40  0.000
Error   20   6467.9    323.4
Total   23  57255.2

S = 17.98   R-Sq = 88.70%   R-Sq(adj) = 87.01%
```

Since the p value for the interaction term is greater than .05, we fail to reject the null hypothesis that there is interaction. After refitting the model without the interaction, we see both dose and treatment are significant.

8.5.3. Results for: EXR_C08_S05_03.mtw

General Linear Model: CHANGE versus MIGRAINE, TREAT

```
Factor     Type   Levels  Values
MIGRAINE   fixed      2   1, 2
TREAT      fixed      2   1, 2

Analysis of Variance for CHANGE, using Adjusted SS for Tests

Source          DF    Seq SS   Adj SS   Adj MS      F      P
MIGRAINE         1    6827.3   7983.7   7983.7  19.98  0.000
TREAT            1     646.9    851.1    851.1   2.13  0.152
MIGRAINE*TREAT   1     567.3    567.3    567.3   1.42  0.240
Error           40   15979.7  15979.7    399.5
Total           43   24021.2

S = 19.9873   R-Sq = 33.48%   R-Sq(adj) = 28.49%
```

General Linear Model: CHANGE versus MIGRAINE, TREAT

```
Factor     Type   Levels  Values
MIGRAINE   fixed      2   1, 2
TREAT      fixed      2   1, 2


Analysis of Variance for CHANGE, using Adjusted SS for Tests

Source     DF    Seq SS    Adj SS   Adj MS      F      P
MIGRAINE    1    6827.3    7453.1   7453.1  18.47  0.000
TREAT       1     646.9     646.9    646.9   1.60  0.213
Error      41   16546.9   16546.9    403.6
Total      43   24021.2


S = 20.0894   R-Sq = 31.12%   R-Sq(adj) = 27.75%
```

Since the *p* value for the interaction term is greater than .05, we fail to reject the null hypothesis that there is interaction. After refitting the model without the interaction, we see treatment remains not significant.

8.5.5.

Factors: Diagnosis of AL (2 levels), Smoking Status (2 levels), Interaction
Response: Pack years, age at first onset of smoking, FEV1, FVC
Extraneous: exercise

Chapter 8 Review Exercises

13. Results for: REV_C08_13.mtw

One-way ANOVA: Count versus Group

```
Source   DF      SS     MS     F      P
Group     4   86.72  21.68  7.04  0.000
Error    70  215.62   3.08
Total    74  302.35

S = 1.755   R-Sq = 28.68%   R-Sq(adj) = 24.61%

                         Individual 95% CIs For Mean Based on
                         Pooled StDev
Level      N   Mean  StDev  --------+---------+---------+---------+-
A          8  6.488  1.767   (---------*---------)
B         18  8.128  1.797                  (------*------)
C         16  7.862  1.640              (-------*------)
D          9  8.233  2.469               (---------*--------)
healthy   24  5.746  1.471  (-----*-----)
                            --------+---------+---------+---------+-
                                 6.0       7.2       8.4       9.6

Pooled StDev = 1.755


Tukey 95% Simultaneous Confidence Intervals
All Pairwise Comparisons among Levels of Group

Individual confidence level = 99.34%

Group = A        subtracted from:

Group     Lower  Center  Upper  --------+---------+---------+---------+-
B        -0.448   1.640  3.729                  (--------*-------)
C        -0.753   1.375  3.503                  (-------*-------)
D        -0.642   1.746  4.134                   (--------*--------)
healthy  -2.748  -0.742  1.265          (------*-------)
                                -------+---------+---------+---------+-
                                    -2.5       0.0       2.5       5.0

Group = B        subtracted from:

Group     Lower  Center  Upper  --------+---------+---------+---------+-
C        -1.954  -0.265  1.423           (------*------)
D        -1.901   0.106  2.112           (-------*-------)
healthy  -3.914  -2.382 -0.850   (-----*------)
                                --------+---------+---------+---------+-
                                    -2.5       0.0       2.5       5.0

Group = C        subtracted from:

Group     Lower  Center  Upper  --------+---------+---------+---------+-
D        -1.677   0.371  2.419            (-------*-------)
healthy  -3.703  -2.117 -0.531   (------*-----)
                                --------+---------+---------+---------+-
                                    -2.5       0.0       2.5       5.0
```

```
Group = D        subtracted from:

Group    Lower  Center   Upper  --------+---------+---------+---------+-
healthy  -4.408  -2.488  -0.567  (-------*-------)
                                 --------+---------+---------+---------+-
                                     -2.5      0.0       2.5       5.0
```

15. Results for: REV_C08_15.mtw

Two-way ANOVA: OUTCOME versus METHOD, SUBJ

```
Source  DF      SS        MS       F      P
METHOD   2  0.05365  0.026827   1.35  0.274
SUBJ    15  8.20068  0.546712  27.55  0.000
Error   30  0.59541  0.019847
Total   47  8.84975

S = 0.1409   R-Sq = 93.27%   R-Sq(adj) = 89.46%
```

V.R. $= 1.35$ $p = .274$ Do not reject H_0 for method.

17. Results for: REV_C08_17.mtw

General Linear Model: AMP versus SMOKE, VEG

```
Factor  Type   Levels  Values
SMOKE   fixed      3   1, 2, 3
VEG     fixed      3   ve1, ve2, ve3


Analysis of Variance for AMP, using Adjusted SS for Tests

Source      DF   Seq SS   Adj SS   Adj MS     F      P
SMOKE        2    78.84   397.66   198.83   3.16  0.052
VEG          2   340.60   861.20   430.60   6.84  0.003
SMOKE*VEG    4   733.10   733.10   183.27   2.91  0.032
Error       43  2706.45  2706.45    62.94
Total       51  3858.98
```

19. Results for: REV_C08_19.mtw

Two-way ANOVA: EMG versus SUBJ, ANGLE

```
Source   DF      SS        MS       F      P
SUBJ     17  14405.2   847.365   12.05  0.000
ANGLE     8   2376.2   297.020    4.23  0.000
Error   136   9560.2    70.296
Total   161  26341.6

S = 8.384   R-Sq = 63.71%   R-Sq(adj) = 57.04%
```

21. Results for: REV_C08_21.mtw

Two-way ANOVA: RESPONSE versus ANIMAL, ANES

```
Source   DF      SS         MS       F       P
ANIMAL    9   0.92652   0.102947   1.11    0.403
ANES      2   1.17091   0.585453   6.32    0.008
Error    18   1.66736   0.092631
Total    29   3.76479
```

```
S = 0.3044   R-Sq = 55.71%   R-Sq(adj) = 28.65%
```

V.R. = 6.320 p = .008

23. Results for: REV_C08_23.mtw

One-way ANOVA: WEIGHT versus GROUP

```
Source   DF      SS        MS      F       P
GROUP     3   1037901   345967   3.12   0.043
Error    27   2995421   110942
Total    30   4033323
```

```
GROUP = A subtracted from:

GROUP   Lower   Center   Upper   ---------+---------+---------+---------+
B       -169.3   302.4   774.1                   (--------*--------)
C       -657.2  -164.9   327.3        (---------*---------)
D       -587.4  -155.1   277.3         (--------*--------)
                                ---------+---------+---------+---------+
                                      -500        0       500      1000


GROUP = B subtracted from:

GROUP   Lower   Center   Upper   ---------+---------+---------+---------+
C       -974.4  -467.3    39.8   (---------*---------)
D       -906.6  -457.4    -8.3   (--------*--------)
                                ---------+---------+---------+---------+
                                      -500        0       500      1000
```

V.R. = 3.1187 p = .043 The sample mean for population D is significantly different from the sample mean for population B. No other differences between sample means are significant.

25. Results for: REV_C08_25.mtw

Two-way ANOVA: VC versus AGEGROUP, OCC

```
Source        DF      SS         MS        F       P
AGEGROUP       2   12.3088   6.15439   29.38   0.000
OCC            3   19.7785   6.59285   31.47   0.000
Interaction    6    8.9489   1.49148    7.12   0.000
Error         48   10.0542   0.20946
Total         59   51.0904
```

```
S = 0.4577   R-Sq = 80.32%   R-Sq(adj) = 75.81%
```

27. 499.5, 9, 166.5, 61.1667, 2.8889, 57.6346, < .005

Source	SS	df	MS	VR	P
Treatments	499.5	3	166.5	57.6346	<.005
Blocks	183.5	3	61.1667		
Error	26.0	9	2.8889		
	709.0	15			

29. **(a)** Completely randomized **(b)** 3 **(c)** 30 **(d)** No, because $1.0438 < 3.35$

31.

Dependent Variable: SERUM

Source	DF	Sum of Squares	Mean Square	F Value	Pr > F
Model	3	216.8571429	72.2857143	26.06	<.0001
Error	24	66.5714286	2.7738095		
Corrected Total	27	283.4285714			

R-Square	Coeff Var	Root MSE	SERUM Mean
0.765121	23.31666	1.665476	7.142857

Pooled St. Dev. = Root MSE = 1.665

$$HSD = 3.90126\sqrt{2.7738095/7} = 2.4458$$

Alpha	0.05
Error Degrees of Freedom	24
Error Mean Square	2.77381
Critical Value of Studentized Range	3.90126
Minimum Significant Difference	2.4558

Comparisons significant at the 0.05 level are indicated by ***.

STATUS Comparison		Difference Between Means	Simultaneous 95% Confidence Limits		
NON	- L	2.5714	0.1156	5.0272	***
NON	- M	4.7143	2.2585	7.1701	***
NON	- H	7.5714	5.1156	10.0272	***
L	- NON	-2.5714	-5.0272	-0.1156	***
L	- M	2.1429	-0.3130	4.5987	
L	- H	5.0000	2.5442	7.4558	***
M	- NON	-4.7143	-7.1701	-2.2585	***
M	- L	-2.1429	-4.5987	0.3130	
M	- H	2.8571	0.4013	5.3130	***
H	- NON	-7.5714	-10.0272	-5.1156	***
H	- L	-5.0000	-7.4558	-2.5442	***
H	- M	-2.8571	-5.3130	-0.4013	***

All differences significant except $\mu_{Light} - \mu_{Moderate}$

33.
Results for: REV_C08_33.mtw

One-way ANOVA: GLUCOSE versus GROUP

```
Source   DF     SS     MS     F     P
GROUP     2   293.1  146.5  2.37  0.117
Error    22  1358.6   61.8
Total    24  1651.7

S = 7.859   R-Sq = 17.74%   R-Sq(adj) = 10.27%
```

V.R. = 2.37 p = .117, Tukey HSD not necessary.

35.   **(a)** One way ANOVA

   (b) Response: Post-Pre training score

   (c) Factors: Groups of years of experience (4 levels).

   (d) Interest in obstetrics, surgical experience

   (e) No carry over effects

   (f) treatment is years of experience $d.f.=3$, total $d.f. = 29$, error $d.f. = 26$.

37.

    (a) Repeated measures

    (b) Response: BMD

    (c) Factors: Time points (6 levels)

    (d) Diet, exercise, calcium intake

    (e) No carry over effects

    (f) time factor $d.f. = 5$, subject factor $d.f. = 25$, total $d.f. = 155$, error $d.f. = 125$.

39.

```
Analysis of Variance for bilirubi
Source      DF       SS       MS       F        P
subject     17    2480.83   145.93   45.57   0.000
time         6      89.09    14.85    4.64   0.000
Error      102     326.65     3.20
Total      125    2896.57
```

41. CR= Compression Ratio

```
Analysis of Variance for C.R.
Source      DF       SS       MS       F        P
Group        4     9092     2273     8.12    0.001
Error       19     5319      280
Total       23    14411
                              Individual 95% CIs For Mean
                              Based on Pooled StDev
Level       N     Mean     StDev   ---+---------+---------+---------+---
Control     6     79.96     5.46                      (-----*-----)
I           4     78.69    21.44                      (------*------)
II          4     47.84    23.74         (------*------)
III         5     43.51    10.43       (-----*------)
IV          5     33.32    20.40   (-----*------)
                                    ---+---------+---------+---------+---
Pooled StDev =    16.73             25        50        75       100
Tukey's pairwise comparisons

     Family error rate = 0.0500
Individual error rate = 0.00728
```

Critical value = 4.25

Intervals for (column level mean) - (row level mean)

	Control	I	II	III
I	-31.19 33.72			
II	-0.34 64.58	-4.70 66.41		
III	6.00 66.89	1.45 68.91	-29.41 38.05	
IV	16.19 77.08	11.64 79.10	-19.21 48.24	-21.61 41.99

43.

Analysis of Variance for BC

Source	DF	SS	MS	F	P
heat	1	0.1602	0.1602	3.95	0.061
chromo	1	0.6717	0.6717	16.55	0.001
Interaction	1	0.0000	0.0000	0.00	0.994
Error	20	0.8119	0.0406		
Total	23	1.6438			

S = 0.2015   R-Sq = 50.61%   R-Sq(adj) = 43.20%

```
                    Individual 95% CIs For Mean Based on
                    Pooled StDev
HEAT      Mean    ---+---------+---------+---------+------
NO      0.612167                   (---------*---------)
YES     0.448750  (---------*----------)
                  ---+---------+---------+---------+------
                   0.36      0.48      0.60      0.72
```

```
                    Individual 95% CIs For Mean Based on
                    Pooled StDev
CHROMO    Mean    ----+---------+---------+---------+-----
NO      0.363167  (-------*-------)
YES     0.697750                    (-------*-------)
                  ----+---------+---------+---------+-----
                    0.30      0.45      0.60      0.75
```

Analysis of Variance for AC

Source	DF	SS	MS	F	P
heat	1	0.0468	0.0468	1.99	0.174
chromo	1	0.4554	0.4554	19.34	0.000
Interaction	1	0.0039	0.0039	0.16	0.690
Error	20	0.4709	0.0235		
Total	23	0.9769			

S = 0.1534   R-Sq = 51.80%   R-Sq(adj) = 44.57%

```
                    Individual 95% CIs For Mean Based on
                    Pooled StDev
HEAT      Mean    -------+---------+---------+---------+--
NO      0.484917                 (------------*------------)
YES     0.396583  (-------------*------------)
                  -------+---------+---------+---------+--
                      0.350     0.420     0.490     0.560


                    Individual 95% CIs For Mean Based on
                    Pooled StDev
CHROMO    Mean    --+---------+---------+---------+-------
NO      0.303000  (------*-------)
YES     0.578500                       (------*-------)
                  --+---------+---------+---------+-------
                    0.24      0.36      0.48      0.60
```

Analysis of Variance for AC/BC

Source	DF	SS	MS	F	P
heat	1	0.04524	0.04524	15.62	0.001
chromo	1	0.00000	0.00000	0.00	1.000
Interaction	1	0.00385	0.00385	1.33	0.262
Error	20	0.05793	0.00290		
Total	23	0.10702			

$S = 0.05382$ $R\text{-Sq} = 45.87\%$ $R\text{-Sq(adj)} = 37.75\%$

```
                    Individual 95% CIs For Mean Based on
                    Pooled StDev
HEAT      Mean    ------+---------+---------+---------+---
NO      0.806833  (-------*-------)
YES     0.893667                     (-------*--------)
                  ------+---------+---------+---------+---
                      0.800     0.840     0.880     0.920


                    Individual 95% CIs For Mean Based on
                    Pooled StDev
CHROMO    Mean    -+---------+---------+---------+--------
NO      0.850250  (--------------*--------------)
YES     0.850250  (--------------*--------------)
                  -+---------+---------+---------+--------
                   0.820     0.840     0.860     0.880
```

45.

```
C.A. = Congruence Angle
Analysis of Variance for C.A.
Source     DF        SS        MS        F        P
Group       3      7598      2533    14.83    0.000
Error      86     14690       171
Total      89     22288
                                  Individual 95% CIs For Mean
                                  Based on Pooled StDev
Level       N      Mean     StDev   -----+---------+---------+---------+-
Lateral    27      6.78     15.10                           (----*----)
Medial     26    -10.81     10.80             (----*----)
Multi      17    -18.29     15.09   (------*-----)
Normal     20     -7.00     10.76           (-----*-----)
                                  -----+---------+---------+---------+-
Pooled StDev =    13.07          -20       -10        0        10

Tukey's pairwise comparisons

     Family error rate = 0.0500
Individual error rate = 0.0103


Critical value = 3.71

Intervals for (column level mean) - (row level mean)

              Lateral     Medial     Multi

   Medial        8.16
                27.01

   Multi        14.46      -3.21
                35.69      18.18

   Normal        3.66     -14.01    -22.60
                23.89       6.39      0.02
```

47. The 6 subjects are tested at 3 different temperatures. It is a repeated measures design.

```
Analysis of Variance for response
Source     DF        SS        MS        F        P
subject     5     25.78      5.16     4.72    0.018
temp        2     30.34     15.17    13.87    0.001
Error      10     10.93      1.09
Total      17     67.06
```

49. Results for: REV_C08_49.mtw

GC = glucose concentration

Two-way ANOVA: GC versus GROUP, SUBJ

```
Source  DF        SS        MS      F      P
GROUP    3    8.3409   2.78030  10.18  0.001
SUBJ     5    8.7735   1.75470   6.43  0.002
Error   15    4.0960   0.27306
Total   23   21.2104

S = 0.5226   R-Sq = 80.69%   R-Sq(adj) = 70.39%
```

```
                       Individual 95% CIs For Mean Based on
                       Pooled StDev
GROUP     Mean    -+---------+---------+---------+--------
A 1    4.01333    (-------*------)
A 2    4.68000            (-------*-------)
B      5.35000                      (------*-------)
C      5.49500                         (------*------)
                  -+---------+---------+---------+--------
                 3.60      4.20      4.80      5.40
```

```
                       Individual 95% CIs For Mean Based on
                       Pooled StDev
SUBJ        Mean    +---------+---------+---------+---------
1.000000  4.87500             (------*------)
2.000000  3.78250   (------*------)
3.000000  4.87250             (------*------)
4.000000  5.68250                    (------*------)
5.000000  5.42750                  (------*------ )
6.000000  4.66750          (------*------)
                    +---------+---------+---------+---------
                   3.20      4.00      4.80      5.60
```

51. Results for: REV_C08_51.mtw

Two-way ANOVA: T3 versus SUBJ, DAY

```
Source  DF        SS        MS      F      P
SUBJ    11    8967.4    815.22   2.55  0.030
DAY      2   12466.2   6233.08  19.50  0.000
Error   22    7033.2    319.69
Total   35   28466.8

S = 17.88   R-Sq = 75.29%   R-Sq(adj) = 60.69%
```

53. Results for: REV_C08_53.mtw

One-way ANOVA: BBL versus GROUP

```
Source  DF    SS    MS     F      P
GROUP    2  4077  2039  3.31  0.090
Error    8  4931   616
Total   10  9008

S = 24.83   R-Sq = 45.26%   R-Sq(adj) = 31.57%


                                  Individual 95% CIs For Mean Based on
                                  Pooled StDev
Level            N   Mean  StDev  ---+---------+---------+---------+------
Control          4  63.50  28.25          (--------*---------)
Hypercarbia      4  50.00  22.69  (---------*--------)
Hyperosmolality  3  98.00  22.27                      (---------*----------)
                                  ---+---------+---------+---------+------
                                    30        60        90       120

Pooled StDev = 24.83


Tukey 95% Simultaneous Confidence Intervals
All Pairwise Comparisons among Levels of GROUP

Individual confidence level = 97.87%


GROUP = Control        subtracted from:

GROUP            Lower   Center  Upper
Hypercarbia     -63.65  -13.50  36.65
Hyperosmolality -19.67   34.50  88.67

GROUP           -------+---------+---------+---------+--
Hypercarbia            (--------*-------)
Hyperosmolality                 (-------*--------)
                -------+---------+---------+---------+--
                     -60        0        60       120


GROUP = Hypercarbia    subtracted from:

GROUP            Lower   Center  Upper
Hyperosmolality  -6.17   48.00  102.17

GROUP           -------+---------+---------+---------+--
Hyperosmolality                 (--------*-------)
                -------+---------+---------+---------+--
                     -60        0        60       120
```

55. Results for: REV_C08_55.mtw

One-way ANOVA: scores versus group

```
Source  DF      SS      MS      F      P
group    2  244.17  122.08  14.50  0.000
Error   38  319.88    8.42
Total   40  564.05

S = 2.901   R-Sq = 43.29%   R-Sq(adj) = 40.30%


                          Individual 95% CIs For Mean Based on
                          Pooled StDev
Level   N    Mean  StDev  ----+---------+---------+---------+-----
1      13  13.231  1.739  (------*-----)
2      14  13.786  2.833    (-----*-----)
3      14  18.643  3.713                       (------*-----)
                          ----+---------+---------+---------+-----
                          12.5      15.0      17.5      20.0

Pooled StDev = 2.901


Tukey 95% Simultaneous Confidence Intervals
All Pairwise Comparisons among Levels of group

Individual confidence level = 98.05%


group = 1 subtracted from:

group  Lower  Center  Upper  ---------+---------+---------+---------+
2     -2.171   0.555  3.281             (-----*------)
3      2.686   5.412  8.138                        (------*-----)
                             ---------+---------+---------+---------+
                                  -4.0      0.0       4.0       8.0


group = 2 subtracted from:

group  Lower  Center  Upper  ---------+---------+---------+---------+
3      2.182   4.857  7.532                        (------*------)
                             ---------+---------+---------+---------+
                                  -4.0      0.0       4.0       8.0
```

57. Results for: REV_C08_57.mtw

One-way ANOVA: PSWQ versus Group

```
Source   DF       SS      MS      F      P
Group     3  16654.9  5551.6  74.11  0.000
Error   115   8614.6    74.9
Total   118  25269.5

S = 8.655   R-Sq = 65.91%   R-Sq(adj) = 65.02%


                               Individual 95% CIs For Mean Based on
                               Pooled StDev
Level         N    Mean   StDev  -----+---------+---------+---------+----
1.000000     15  62.933   8.556                           (---*---)
2.000000     30  38.333   7.494  (--*--)
3.000000     19  64.158  10.259                      (---*---)
4.000000     55  66.536   8.678                           (--*-)
                               -----+---------+---------+---------+----
                                   40        50        60        70

Pooled StDev = 8.655


Tukey 95% Simultaneous Confidence Intervals
All Pairwise Comparisons among Levels of Group

Individual confidence level = 98.97%


Group = 1.000000 subtracted from:

Group        Lower   Center    Upper  -------+---------+---------+---------+--
2.000000   -31.741  -24.600  -17.459  (---*--)
3.000000    -6.575    1.225    9.025                 (---*---)
4.000000    -2.975    3.603   10.181                 (--*--)
                                      -------+---------+---------+---------+--
                                           -20         0        20        40


Group = 2.000000 subtracted from:

Group       Lower  Center   Upper  -------+---------+---------+---------+--
3.000000   19.203  25.825  32.446                          (--*--)
4.000000   23.077  28.203  33.329                           (-*--)
                                   -------+---------+---------+---------+--
                                        -20         0        20        40


Group = 3.000000 subtracted from:

Group       Lower  Center  Upper  -------+---------+---------+---------+--
4.000000   -3.631   2.378  8.388                  (--*--)
                                  -------+---------+---------+---------+--
                                       -20         0        20        40
```

59. Results for: REV_C08_59.mtw

One-way ANOVA: AGE versus GROUP

```
Source   DF       SS      MS      F       P
GROUP     2   16323.2  8161.6  139.79  0.000
Error   189   11034.7    58.4
Total   191   27357.9

S = 7.641   R-Sq = 59.67%   R-Sq(adj) = 59.24%


                            Individual 95% CIs For Mean Based on
                            Pooled StDev
Level      N    Mean  StDev  --+---------+---------+---------+-------
Daughter  50  49.420  7.508  (--*--)
Husband   65  71.985  7.516                                   (--*--)
Wife      77  68.649  7.828                             (-*--)
                            --+---------+---------+---------+-------
                            49.0      56.0      63.0      70.0

Pooled StDev = 7.641


Tukey 95% Simultaneous Confidence Intervals
All Pairwise Comparisons among Levels of GROUP

Individual confidence level = 98.08%


GROUP = Daughter subtracted from:

GROUP    Lower   Center   Upper  ------+---------+---------+---------+---
Husband  19.170  22.565  25.959                        (---*--)
Wife     15.952  19.229  22.507                      (--*---)
                                 ------+---------+---------+---------+---
                                     0        10        20        30


GROUP = Husband  subtracted from:

GROUP    Lower   Center   Upper  ------+---------+---------+---------+---
Wife     -6.375  -3.335  -0.296  (--*--)
                                 ------+---------+---------+---------+---
                                     0        10        20        30
```

61. Results for: REV_C08_61.mtw

SAP = serum alkaline phosphatase level

One-way ANOVA: SAP versus GRADE

```
Source  DF      SS     MS     F      P
GRADE    2   36181  18091  5.55  0.009
Error   29   94560   3261
Total   31  130742

S = 57.10   R-Sq = 27.67%   R-Sq(adj) = 22.69%


                              Individual 95% CIs For Mean Based on
                              Pooled StDev
Level   N    Mean   StDev    +---------+---------+---------+---------
I       9  118.00   61.85    (--------*---------)
II      8  143.63   55.90          (---------*---------)
III    15  194.80   54.82                        (-------*------)
                             +---------+---------+---------+---------
                             80       120       160       200

Pooled StDev = 57.10


Tukey 95% Simultaneous Confidence Intervals
All Pairwise Comparisons among Levels of GRADE

Individual confidence level = 98.03%


GRADE = I   subtracted from:

GRADE  Lower  Center  Upper   ------+---------+---------+---------+---
II    -42.85   25.63  94.10         (---------*--------)
III    17.38   76.80 136.22               (-------*------)
                             ------+---------+---------+---------+---
                                  -70        0        70       140


GRADE = II  subtracted from:

GRADE  Lower  Center  Upper   ------+---------+---------+---------+---
III   -10.52   51.18 112.87               (--------*-------)
                             ------+---------+---------+---------+---
                                  -70        0        70       140
```

63. Results for: REV_C08_63.mtw

One-way ANOVA: HEMA versus GROUP

```
Source  DF     SS     MS      F      P
GROUP    2   817.5  408.8  20.26  0.000
Error   27   544.8   20.2
Total   29  1362.3

S = 4.492   R-Sq = 60.01%   R-Sq(adj) = 57.05%

                              Individual 95% CIs For Mean Based on
                              Pooled StDev
Level        N    Mean   StDev   -+---------+---------+---------+--------
Sham        10  38.200   2.573   (----*----)
Treated     15  40.200   5.348       (---*---)
Untreated    5  53.200   4.604                             (------*------)
                              -+---------+---------+---------+--------
                              36.0      42.0      48.0      54.0

Pooled StDev = 4.492

Tukey 95% Simultaneous Confidence Intervals
All Pairwise Comparisons among Levels of GROUP

Individual confidence level = 98.04%

GROUP = Sham      subtracted from:

GROUP      Lower  Center   Upper  ---------+---------+---------+---------+
Treated   -2.551   2.000   6.551            (----*----)
Untreated  8.894  15.000  21.106                           (-----*-----)
                              ---------+---------+---------+---------+
                                     -10        0        10       20

GROUP = Treated   subtracted from:

GROUP      Lower  Center   Upper  ---------+---------+---------+---------+
Untreated  7.243  13.000  18.757                         (-----*-----)
                              ---------+---------+---------+---------+
                                     -10        0        10       20
```

65. **Results for: REV_C08_65.mtw**

One-way ANOVA: RESPONSE versus TREAT

Both = rhIGF-I + rhGH

```
Source  DF      SS     MS     F      P
TREAT    3   4.148  1.383  1.39  0.282
Error   16  15.898  0.994
Total   19  20.046

S = 0.9968   R-Sq = 20.69%   R-Sq(adj) = 5.82%


                                 Individual 95% CIs For Mean Based on
                                 Pooled StDev
Level     N    Mean   StDev   --------+---------+---------+---------+-
Both      5  11.520   0.653                   (--------*---------)
rhGH      5  11.250   0.570                (--------*---------)
rhIGF-I   6  10.800   1.418             (--------*--------)
Saline    4  10.250   0.971   (---------*----------)
                              --------+---------+---------+---------+-
                                  10.0      11.0      12.0      13.0

Pooled StDev = 0.997
```

Chapter 9

9.3.1. (a) Direct, **(b)** Direct, **(c)** Inverse

9.3.3. Results for: EXR_C09_S03_03.mtw

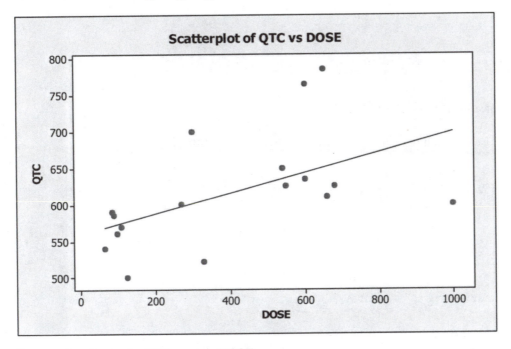

Regression Analysis: QTC versus DOSE

```
The regression equation is
QTC = 560 + 0.140 DOSE
```

9.3.5. $\hat{y} = 68.6 - 19.5x$

9.3.7. Results for: EXR_C09_S03_07.mtw

Regression Analysis: INVCYS versus DTPA

```
The regression equation is
INVCYS = 0.193 + 0.00628 DTPA
```

9.4.1. Results for: EXR_C09_S03_03.mtw

```
Predictor        Coef      SE Coef          T          P
Constant        559.90       29.13       19.22      0.000
Meth Dos       0.13989      0.06033        2.32      0.035

S = 68.28       R-Sq = 26.4%     R-Sq(adj) = 21.5%

Analysis of Variance

Source           DF           SS          MS          F          P
Regression        1        25063       25063       5.38      0.035
Residual Error   15        69923        4662
Total            16        94986
```

Confidence interval for β: .011, .268

9.4.3. Use data from Exercise 9.3.5. Results obtained from MINITAB

```
Predictor        Coef      SE Coef          T          P
Constant         68.64       16.68        4.12      0.006
Cmax w/        -19.529        4.375       -4.46      0.004

S = 18.87       R-Sq = 76.9%     R-Sq(adj) = 73.0%

Analysis of Variance

Source           DF           SS          MS          F          P
Regression        1       7098.4      7098.4      19.93      0.004
Residual Error    6       2137.4       356.2
Total             7       9235.9
```

Confidence interval for β: -30.23, -8.82

9.4.5. Use data from Exercise 9.3.7. Results obtained from MINITAB

```
Predictor        Coef      SE Coef          T          P
Constant       0.19290      0.04849        3.98      0.001
DTPA GFR      0.006279     0.001059        5.93      0.000

S = 0.09159     R-Sq = 58.5%     R-Sq(adj) = 56.8%

Analysis of Variance

Source           DF           SS          MS          F          P
Regression        1      0.29509     0.29509      35.18      0.000
Residual Error   25      0.20972     0.00839
Total            26      0.50481
```

Confidence interval for β: 0.0041, 0.0085

9.5.1. **(a)** 580.6, 651.2   **(b)** 466.1, 765.6

9.5.3. **(a)** -30.42, 5.22   **(b)** -62.11, 36.92

9.5.5. **(a)** 0.3727, 0.4526   **(b)** 0.2199, 0.6055

9.7.1 $r = .466$, $t = 2.23$, $p = .038$, $.030 < ? < .775$

The correlation between age and bilirubin levels is statistically significant.

9.7.3. $r = -.812$, $t = -3.11$, $p = .027$, $-1 < ? < -.152$

The correlation between AUC levels when taking water and when taking grapefruit juice is statistically significant.

9.7.5 $r = -.531$, $t = -3.31$, $p = .003$, $-.770 < ? < -.211$

The correlation between the partial pressure of arterial oxygen and the partial pressure of arterial carbon dioxide is statistically significant.

Chapter 9 Review Exercises

17. Results for: REV_C09_17.mtw

Regression Analysis: BOARD versus AVG

```
The regression equation is
BOARD = - 191 + 4.68 AVG


Predictor      Coef   SE Coef       T       P
Constant    -191.03     22.93   -8.33   0.000
AVG          4.6815    0.2727   17.17   0.000

S = 12.4918   R-Sq = 77.2%   R-Sq(adj) = 76.9%

Analysis of Variance

Source            DF      SS      MS       F       P
Regression         1   45998   45998  294.77   0.000
Residual Error    87   13576     156
Total             88   59574


Unusual Observations

Obs    AVG   BOARD     Fit   SE Fit   Residual   St Resid
  1   95.7  257.00  257.13     3.47      -0.13     -0.01 X
 24   86.9  187.00  215.60     1.54     -28.60     -2.31R
 37   84.6  176.00  204.93     1.33     -28.93     -2.33R
 43   84.1  229.00  202.82     1.32      26.18      2.11R
 48   83.9  176.00  201.84     1.32     -25.84     -2.08R
 55   82.8  169.00  196.69     1.36     -27.69     -2.23R
 65   81.5  230.00  190.56     1.48      39.44      3.18R
 68   80.9  160.00  187.80     1.56     -27.80     -2.24R
 89   70.3  159.00  138.27     3.94      20.73      1.75 X

R denotes an observation with a large standardized residual.
X denotes an observation whose X value gives it large influence.
```

19. Results for: REV_C09_19.mtw

Regression Analysis: TIME versus PROBLEMS

```
The regression equation is
TIME = 12.6 + 1.80 PROBLEMS


Predictor     Coef   SE Coef      T       P
Constant    12.641     2.133   5.93   0.000
PROBLEMS    1.8045    0.5585   3.23   0.005


S = 7.08098   R-Sq = 38.0%   R-Sq(adj) = 34.4%


Analysis of Variance

Source          DF        SS        MS       F       P
Regression       1    523.41    523.41   10.44   0.005
Residual Error  17    852.38     50.14
Total           18   1375.79
```

21. Results for: REV_C09_21.mtw

Regression Analysis: B versus A

```
The regression equation is
B = 1.28 + 0.851 A


Predictor     Coef   SE Coef      T       P
Constant    1.2763    0.3935   3.24   0.006
A           0.8513    0.1601   5.32   0.000


S = 0.240908   R-Sq = 68.5%   R-Sq(adj) = 66.1%


Analysis of Variance

Source          DF       SS       MS       F       P
Regression       1   1.6418   1.6418   28.29   0.000
Residual Error  13   0.7545   0.0580
Total           14   2.3963
```

23. Results for: REV_C09_23.mtw

Regression Analysis: GLUCOSE versus WEIGHT

```
The regression equation is
GLUCOSE = 61.9 + 0.510 WEIGHT


Predictor     Coef   SE Coef     T       P
Constant     61.88     19.19   3.22   0.006
WEIGHT      0.5098    0.2462   2.07   0.057


S = 9.27608   R-Sq = 23.4%   R-Sq(adj) = 18.0%


Analysis of Variance

Source         DF       SS       MS      F       P
Regression      1   368.80   368.80   4.29   0.057
Residual Error 14  1204.64    86.05
Total          15  1573.44
```

$r = .484$, CI: (-.03, .79); predicted glucose when weight = 95 is 110.30.
The 95% prediction interval is (87.7796, 132.827)

25. Results for: REV_C09_25.mtw

Regression Analysis: TEMP versus TIME

```
The regression equation is
TEMP = 37.5 + 0.0798 TIME


Predictor       Coef    SE Coef       T       P
Constant     37.4564     0.3959   94.61   0.000
TIME        0.079849   0.009092    8.78   0.000


S = 0.330335   R-Sq = 90.6%   R-Sq(adj) = 89.4%


Analysis of Variance

Source         DF      SS      MS      F       P
Regression      1  8.4160  8.4160  77.13   0.000
Residual Error  8  0.8730  0.1091
Total           9  9.2890
```

$r = .952$, CI: (.910, 1.0); predicted Temp when Time = 50 is 41.4488.

The 95% prediction interval is (40.6324, 42.2651)

29. Results for: REV_C09_29.mtw

Regression Analysis: A versus B

```
The regression equation is
A = 570 + 0.429 B

Predictor      Coef   SE Coef     T      P
Constant      569.8     141.2   4.03   0.000
B           0.42927   0.04353   9.86   0.000

S = 941.560    R-Sq = 54.0%   R-Sq(adj) = 53.4%

Analysis of Variance

Source          DF         SS         MS       F      P
Regression       1   86208485   86208485   97.24   0.000
Residual Error  83   73582364     886535
Total           84  159790850

Unusual Observations

Obs     B      A    Fit   SE Fit   Residual   St Resid
 32   727   3900    882      122       3018      3.23R
 33   745   4050    890      121       3160      3.38R
 69  4300   4960   2416      136       2544      2.73R
 70  4560   7180   2527      144       4653      5.00R
 76  6230   1260   3244      201      -1984     -2.16R
 83  7800   4910   3918      263        992      1.10 X
 84  8890   4080   4386      307       -306     -0.34 X
 85  9930   3840   4832      350       -992     -1.14 X
```

R denotes an observation with a large standardized residual.
X denotes an observation whose X value gives it large influence.

Performing regression when B < 1000

Regression Analysis: A versus B

```
The regression equation is
A = - 99.6 + 1.5504 B

Predictor      Coef   SE Coef     T      P
Constant      -99.6     247.2  -0.40   0.689
B            1.5504    0.4475   3.46   0.001

S = 733.509    R-Sq = 24.5%   R-Sq(adj) = 22.5%

Analysis of Variance

Source          DF         SS        MS       F      P
Regression       1    6457724   6457724   12.00   0.001
Residual Error  37   19907328    538036
Total           38   26365052
```

```
Unusual Observations

Obs    B      A    Fit   SE Fit   Residual   St Resid
 32   727   3900   1028     159       2872      4.01R
 33   745   4050   1055     165       2995      4.19R

R denotes an observation with a large standardized residual.
```

31. Results for: REV_C09_31.mtw

Regression Analysis: Y versus X

```
The regression equation is
Y = 45.0 + 0.867 X

Predictor     Coef   SE Coef       T      P
Constant     44.99     33.54    1.34   0.193
X          0.86738   0.07644   11.35   0.000

S = 102.889   R-Sq = 84.8%   R-Sq(adj) = 84.2%

Analysis of Variance

Source           DF        SS        MS        F      P
Regression        1   1362983   1362983   128.75   0.000
Residual Error   23    243481     10586
Total            24   1606464
```

Correlations: X, Y

```
Pearson correlation of X and Y = 0.921
P-Value = 0.000
```

33. Results for: REV_C09_33.mtw

Regression Analysis: S versus DBS

```
The regression equation is
S = - 1.26 + 2.10 DBS

Predictor     Coef   SE Coef       T      P
Constant    -1.263     3.019   -0.42   0.680
DBS         2.0970    0.1435   14.62   0.000


S = 8.31594   R-Sq = 90.3%   R-Sq(adj) = 89.9%

Analysis of Variance

Source           DF      SS      MS        F      P
Regression        1   14776   14776   213.66   0.000
Residual Error   23    1591      69
Total            24   16366
```

Unusual Observations

```
Obs    DBS        S      Fit  SE Fit  Residual  St Resid
  1   23.0    64.00    46.97    1.84     17.03     2.10R
  4   53.0   103.00   109.88    5.35     -6.88    -1.08 X
 14   13.0     9.00    26.00    1.79    -17.00    -2.09R
```

R denotes an observation with a large standardized residual.
X denotes an observation whose X value gives it large influence.

Correlations: S, DBS

Pearson correlation of S and DBS = 0.950
P-Value = 0.000

35. Results for: REV_C09_35.mtw

Regression Analysis: LOGPCAL versus PCU

The regression equation is
LOGPCAL = 2.06 + 0.0559 PCU

```
Predictor     Coef   SE Coef     T      P
Constant    2.0603    0.3007   6.85  0.000
PCU        0.05593   0.01631   3.43  0.001
```

S = 0.387317   R-Sq = 16.4%   R-Sq(adj) = 15.0%

Analysis of Variance

```
Source           DF       SS      MS      F      P
Regression        1   1.7648  1.7648  11.76  0.001
Residual Error   60   9.0009  0.1500
Total            61  10.7657
```

Unusual Observations

```
Obs    PCU  LOGPCAL     Fit  SE Fit  Residual  St Resid
  3   27.4   3.2918  3.5938  0.1583   -0.3020    -0.85 X
  8   19.0   4.0200  3.1246  0.0510    0.8954     2.33R
  9   16.4   4.4125  2.9781  0.0572    1.4344     3.74R
 15   25.0   3.9975  3.4585  0.1214    0.5390     1.47 X
 19   18.1   3.9394  3.0732  0.0492    0.8662     2.25R
 58    9.5   2.7143  2.5911  0.1502    0.1232     0.35 X
```

R denotes an observation with a large standardized residual.
X denotes an observation whose X value gives it large influence.

Pearson correlation of PCu and log y = 0.405
P-Value = 0.001

37. Results for: REV_C09_37.mtw

Regression Analysis: LNSKIN versus LNIGE

```
The regression equation is
LNSKIN = - 0.141 - 1.33 LNIGE


Predictor      Coef   SE Coef       T      P
Constant    -0.1413    0.2267   -0.62  0.540
LNIGE       -1.3286    0.1242  -10.69  0.000


S = 1.08635   R-Sq = 84.5%   R-Sq(adj) = 83.7%


Analysis of Variance

Source          DF      SS      MS       F      P
Regression       1  134.97  134.97  114.36  0.000
Residual Error  21   24.78    1.18
Total           22  159.75


Unusual Observations

Obs  LNIGE  LNSKIN    Fit  SE Fit  Residual  St Resid
  9   0.81   1.466  -1.219   0.244     2.685     2.54R

R denotes an observation with a large standardized residual.
```

Correlations: LNIGE, LNSKIN

```
Pearson correlation of LNIGE and LNSKIN = -0.919
P-Value = 0.000
```

39. Normotensive

C6=C4-C5, C7=(C4+C5)/2, C8=C2-C3, C9=(C2+C3)/2

```
The regression equation is
C6 = 4.2 + 0.106 C7

Predictor        Coef    SE Coef       T      P
Constant         4.19      17.30    0.24  0.811
C7             0.1060     0.1590    0.67  0.512

S = 5.251       R-Sq = 2.0%      R-Sq(adj) = 0.0%


Pearson correlation of C6 and C7 = 0.141
P-Value = 0.512
```

```
The regression equation is
C8 = 0.2 + 0.268 C9

Predictor        Coef      SE Coef           T         P
Constant         0.25        18.53        0.01     0.989
C9             0.2682       0.2932        0.91     0.370

S = 5.736       R-Sq = 3.7%      R-Sq(adj) = 0.0%

Pearson correlation of C8 and C9 = 0.191
P-Value = 0.370
```

Preclamptic
```
The regression equation is
C6 = 57.9 - 0.363 C7

Predictor        Coef      SE Coef           T         P
Constant        57.89        17.10        3.39     0.003
C7            -0.3625       0.1273       -2.85     0.009

S = 7.109       R-Sq = 26.9%      R-Sq(adj) = 23.6%

Pearson correlation of C6 and C7 = -0.519
P-Value = 0.009


The regression equation is
C8 = 54.4 - 0.540 C9

Predictor        Coef      SE Coef           T         P
Constant       54.377        9.771        5.56     0.000
C9            -0.5403       0.1154       -4.68     0.000

S = 5.787       R-Sq = 49.9%      R-Sq(adj) = 47.6%


Pearson correlation of C8 and C9 = -0.707
P-Value = 0.000
```

41. Results for: REV_C09_41.mtw

Regression Analysis: LBMD versus ABMD

```
The regression equation is
LBMD = 0.131 + 0.511 ABMD


Predictor     Coef   SE Coef      T       P
Constant   0.13097   0.05413   2.42   0.018
ABMD       0.51056   0.05935   8.60   0.000


S = 0.0918806   R-Sq = 53.6%   R-Sq(adj) = 52.9%

Analysis of Variance

Source           DF        SS        MS       F       P
Regression        1   0.62478   0.62478   74.01   0.000
Residual Error   64   0.54029   0.00844
Total            65   1.16507
```

```
Unusual Observations

Obs   ABMD    LBMD    Fit   SE Fit  Residual  St Resid
 37   0.70   0.1940  0.4904  0.0159  -0.2964   -3.28R
 52   1.41   0.7660  0.8514  0.0328  -0.0854   -0.99 X
 64   1.11   0.4580  0.6962  0.0171  -0.2382   -2.64R
 65   1.58   0.9750  0.9392  0.0425   0.0358    0.44 X
```

R denotes an observation with a large standardized residual.
X denotes an observation whose X value gives it large influence.

Correlations: ABMD, LBMD

```
Pearson correlation of ABMD and LBMD = 0.732
P-Value = 0.000
```

43. Results for: REV_C09_43.mtw

WL, V02

```
The regression equation is
wl = 0.01 + 0.262 vo2

Predictor       Coef     SE Coef        T        P
Constant       0.013       1.308     0.01    0.992
vo2          0.26237     0.07233     3.63    0.003

S = 1.835      R-Sq = 52.3%    R-Sq(adj) = 48.3%

Pearson correlation of wl and vo2 = 0.723
P-Value = 0.003
```

WL, AT

```
The regression equation is
wl = 0.75 + 0.367 at

Predictor       Coef     SE Coef        T        P
Constant       0.752       1.761     0.43    0.677
at            0.3668      0.1660     2.21    0.047

S = 2.241      R-Sq = 28.9%    R-Sq(adj) = 23.0%

Pearson correlation of wl and at = 0.538
P-Value = 0.047
```

WL, ET

```
The regression equation is
wl = 0.74 + 0.00637 et

Predictor       Coef     SE Coef        T        P
Constant       0.739       1.173     0.63    0.541
et          0.006375    0.001840     3.46    0.005

S = 1.879      R-Sq = 50.0%    R-Sq(adj) = 45.8%

Pearson correlation of wl and et = 0.707
P-Value = 0.005
```

45. Results for: REV_C09_45.mtw

Regression Analysis: CLF versus CLER

```
The regression equation is
CLF = 19.4 + 0.893 CLER


Predictor      Coef   SE Coef       T       P
Constant     19.393     4.496    4.31   0.000
CLER        0.89250   0.05671   15.74   0.000


S = 28.2040   R-Sq = 59.3%   R-Sq(adj) = 59.1%


Analysis of Variance

Source           DF       SS       MS        F       P
Regression        1   197013   197013   247.67   0.000
Residual Error  170   135229      795
Total           171   332242


Unusual Observations

Obs   CLER     CLF     Fit   SE Fit   Residual   St Resid
  3    100  165.00  108.64     2.76      56.36       2.01R
 15     88  165.00   97.93     2.39      67.07       2.39R
 17     92  159.00  101.50     2.50      57.50       2.05R
 28     96   47.00  105.07     2.62     -58.07      -2.07R
 30    122   67.00  128.28     3.67     -61.28      -2.19R
 53    110   26.00  117.57     3.14     -91.57      -3.27R
 73     85  163.00   95.08     2.32      67.92       2.42R
103     94   39.10  103.02     2.55     -63.92      -2.28R
147    121  203.00  127.39     3.62      75.61       2.70R
155    110  221.00  117.57     3.14     103.43       3.69R
159    115  201.00  122.03     3.35      78.97       2.82R
162    169  162.00  170.23     6.03      -8.23      -0.30 X
```

R denotes an observation with a large standardized residual.
X denotes an observation whose X value gives it large influence.

Correlations: CLF, CLER

```
Pearson correlation of CLF and CLER = 0.770
P-Value = 0.000
```

Chapter 10

10.3.1 Results for: EXR_C10_S03_01.mtw

Regression Analysis: Y versus X1, X2

```
The regression equation is
Y = - 31.4 + 0.473 X1 + 1.07 X2


Predictor      Coef  SE Coef       T      P
Constant    -31.425    6.147   -5.11  0.000
X1          0.47317  0.06117    7.74  0.000
X2          1.07117  0.06280   17.06  0.000


S = 2.06379   R-Sq = 92.0%   R-Sq(adj) = 91.5%


Analysis of Variance

Source          DF       SS      MS       F      P
Regression       2  1576.99  788.50  185.13  0.000
Residual Error  32   136.30    4.26
Total           34  1713.29


Source  DF   Seq SS
X1       1   337.69
X2       1  1239.30


Unusual Observations

Obs  X1      Y     Fit  SE Fit  Residual  St Resid
 15  97  65.640  59.367   0.573     6.273     3.16R

R denotes an observation with a large standardized residual.
```

10.3.3. Results for: EXR_C10_S03_03.mtw

Regression Analysis: Y versus X1, X2

```
The regression equation is
Y = 13.4 + 4.02 X1 + 2.81 X2


Predictor   Coef  SE Coef     T      P
Constant   13.45    13.23  1.02  0.343
X1         4.017    1.071  3.75  0.007
X2         2.812    1.379  2.04  0.081


S = 5.66569   R-Sq = 66.8%   R-Sq(adj) = 57.3%
```

```
Analysis of Variance

Source          DF      SS      MS      F       P
Regression       2   452.56  226.28   7.05   0.021
Residual Error   7   224.70   32.10
Total            9   677.26


Source   DF   Seq SS
X1        1   319.03
X2        1   133.53
```

10.3.5. Results for: EXR_C10_S03_05.mtw

Regression Analysis: Y versus X1, X2

```
The regression equation is
Y = - 422 + 11.2 X1 - 0.630 X2


Predictor      Coef   SE Coef      T       P
Constant      -422.0    339.8   -1.24   0.227
X1            11.166    3.655    3.05   0.006
X2           -0.6303   0.9383   -0.67   0.509


S = 41.7145   R-Sq = 30.8%   R-Sq(adj) = 24.5%


Analysis of Variance

Source          DF      SS     MS      F       P
Regression       2   17018   8509   4.89   0.017
Residual Error  22   38282   1740
Total           24   55300


Source   DF   Seq SS
X1        1   16232
X2        1     785
```

10.4.1.
Dependent Variable: Y

Source	DF	Sum of Squares	Mean Square	F Value	Pr > F
Model	2	1576.990115	788.495057	185.13	<.0001
Error	32	136.295160	4.259224		
Corrected Total	34	1713.285274			

R-Square	Coeff Var	Root MSE	Y Mean
0.920448	4.026837	2.063789	51.25086

Parameter	Estimate	Standard Error	t Value	Pr > |t|	95% Confidence Limits	
Intercept	-31.42479845	6.14746676	-5.11	<.0001	-43.94677847	-18.90281843
X1	0.47317427	0.06116530	7.74	<.0001	0.34858463	0.59776392
X2	1.07117247	0.06279667	17.06	<.0001	0.94325985	1.19908509

10.4.3.
Dependent Variable: Y

Source	DF	Sum of Squares	Mean Square	F Value	Pr > F
Model	2	452.5637544	226.2818772	7.05	0.0210
Error	7	224.7002456	32.1000351		
Corrected Total	9	677.2640000			

R-Square	Coeff Var	Root MSE	Y Mean
0.668224	9.911983	5.665689	57.16000

Parameter	Estimate	Standard Error	t Value	Pr > |t|	95% Confidence Limits	
Intercept	13.44922863	13.23155592	1.02	0.3433	-17.83842937	44.73688663
X1	4.01679785	1.07135885	3.75	0.0072	1.48343674	6.55015896
X2	2.81175439	1.37858975	2.04	0.0808	-0.44809236	6.07160114

10.4.5.
Dependent Variable: Y

Source	DF	Sum of Squares	Mean Square	F Value	Pr > F
Model	2	17017.78484	8508.89242	4.89	0.0175
Error	22	38282.21516	1740.10069		
Corrected Total	24	55300.00000			

R-Square	Coeff Var	Root MSE	Y Mean
0.307736	7.768066	41.71451	537.0000

Parameter	Estimate	Standard Error	t Value	Pr > |t|	95% Confidence Limits	
Intercept	-421.9967138	339.7619898	-1.24	0.2273	-1126.619954	282.6265263
X1	11.1661344	3.6552338	3.05	0.0058	3.5856435	18.7466253
X2	-0.6303187	0.9382608	-0.67	0.5087	-2.5761524	1.3155151

10.5.1. CI: 50.289, 51.747 PI: 46.751, 55.284

10.5.3. CI: 44.22, 56.59 PI: 35.64, 65.17

10.5.5. CI: 514.31, 550.75 PI: 444.12, 620.94

10.6.1.

(a) Pairwise correlations:

Correlations: Y, X1, X2, X3

```
        Y       X1      X2
X1   0.360
     0.022

X2   0.532   0.303
     0.000   0.058

X3   0.202   0.674   0.430
     0.211   0.000   0.006

Cell Contents: Pearson correlation
               P-Value
```

(b)
```
The regression equation is
Y = 27.8 + 62.6 X1 + 0.0480 X2 - 0.0623 X3


Predictor       Coef  SE Coef      T      P
Constant       27.80    12.91   2.15  0.038
X1             62.58    28.18   2.22  0.033
X2           0.04801  0.01303   3.68  0.001
X3          -0.06229  0.03956  -1.57  0.124


S = 54.0764   R-Sq = 37.0%   R-Sq(adj) = 31.8%


Analysis of Variance

Source          DF      SS     MS      F      P
Regression       3   61892  20631   7.06  0.001
Residual Error  36  105273   2924
Total           39  167165
```

$R = .370, F = 7.06, p = .001$

(c) $r_{y1.23} = .3472, r_{y2.13} = .5232, r_{y3.12} = -.2538$

(d) $r_{12.y3} = -.1660$ **(e)** $r_{13.y2} = .6615$ **(f)** $r_{23.y1} = .3969$

10.6.3.

Model Summary

Model	R	R Square	Adjusted R Square	Std. Error of the Estimate
1	.952[a]	.906	.890	4.161184553

a. Predictors: (Constant), X2, X1

ANOVA[b]

Model		Sum of Squares	df	Mean Square	F	Sig.
1	Regression	1996.084	2	998.042	57.639	.000[a]
	Residual	207.785	12	17.315		
	Total	2203.869	14			

a. Predictors: (Constant), X2, X1

b. Dependent Variable: Y

(b) and (c)

```
- - -   P A R T I A L   C O R R E L A T I O N   C O E F F I C I E N T S   - - -

Controlling for..    X2

                   Y          X1

Y              1.0000        .9268
              (     0)     (    12)
              P=  .        P=  .000


X1              .9268      1.0000
              (    12)     (     0)
              P=  .000     P=  .

- - -   P A R T I A L   C O R R E L A T I O N   C O E F F I C I E N T S   - - -

Controlling for..    X1

                   Y          X2

Y              1.0000        .3784
              (     0)     (    12)
              P=  .        P=  .182


X2              .3784      1.0000
              (    12)     (     0)
              P=  .182     P=  .
```

```
- - -  P A R T I A L   C O R R E L A T I O N   C O E F F I C I E N T S  - - -
```

Controlling for..   Y

```
                    X2              X1

X2               1.0000          -.1788
                (    0)          (   12)
                P= .            P= .541

X1              -.1788           1.0000
                (   12)          (    0)
                P= .541          P= .
```

$r_{y1.2} = .9268, t = 8.549, p < .01; r_{y2.1} = .3785, t = 1.417, .20 > p > .10;$

$r_{12.y} = -.1788, t = -.630, p > .20$

Review Exercises

7. Results for: REV_C10_07.mtw

```
S = 11.4569    R-Sq = 12.2%    R-Sq(adj) = 0.0%
```

Analysis of Variance

```
Source             DF      SS      MS      F       P
Regression          2   219.3   109.6   0.84   0.458
Residual Error     12  1575.1   131.3
Total              14  1794.4
```

$R = .349, F = .84\ (p = .458)$

9. Results for: REV_C10_09.mtw

Regression Analysis: Y versus X1, X2

The regression equation is
Y = 11.4 + 1.26 X1 + 3.11 X2

```
Predictor    Coef  SE Coef       T       P
Constant   11.419    2.761    4.14   0.001
X1         1.2598   0.2032    6.20   0.000
X2         3.1067   0.2981   10.42   0.000

S = 3.63755    R-Sq = 92.0%    R-Sq(adj) = 90.7%
```

```
Analysis of Variance

Source           DF       SS       MS       F       P
Regression        2  1826.95   913.48   69.04   0.000
Residual Error   12   158.78    13.23
Total            14  1985.73
```

$$\hat{y} = 11.419 + 1.2598(10) + 3.1067(5) = 39.55$$

11. Results for: REV_C10_11.mtw

Regression Analysis: Y versus X1, X2, X3, X4

```
The regression equation is
Y = - 127 + 0.176 X1 - 1.56 X2 + 1.57 X3 + 1.63 X4


Predictor      Coef   SE Coef       T       P
Constant    -126.51     32.28   -3.92   0.003
X1          0.17629   0.04009    4.40   0.001
X2           -1.563     2.012   -0.78   0.455
X3           1.5745    0.4457    3.53   0.005
X4           1.6293    0.6287    2.59   0.027


S = 24.0311   R-Sq = 84.2%   R-Sq(adj) = 77.9%


Analysis of Variance

Source           DF       SS       MS       F       P
Regression        4  30873.5   7718.4   13.37   0.001
Residual Error   10   5774.9    577.5
Total            14  36648.4
```

$$R = \sqrt{.842} = .918$$

13.

(a) Correlation

(b) Log plasma adiponectin levels

(c) Age and glomerular filtration rate

(d) Both correlations were not significant

(h) Subjects with end stage renal disease

15.

(a) Correlation

(b) Static inspiratory mouth pressure

(c) Forced expiratory volume, peak expiratory flow, maximal inspiratory flow

(d) Both correlations were not significant

(h) Boys and girls ages 7-14

17. Correlations (Pearson)

	X1	X2	X3	X4	X5	X6	X7	X8	X9	X10	X11	X12	X13
X1	1.0000	0.7366	-0.1091	0.7598	0.5564	0.0397	-0.2912	0.5697	0.5553	0.3448	-0.4672	-0.2496	-0.2711
X2	0.7366	1.0000	0.2437	0.6977	0.6075	-0.2132	-0.2893	0.6585	0.5660	0.5085	-0.3995	-0.2601	-0.3050
X3	-0.1091	0.2437	1.0000	0.3164	0.2732	-0.1357	-0.0930	0.2267	0.1461	0.4195	-0.2235	-0.1776	-0.3803
X4	0.7598	0.6977	0.3164	1.0000	0.7601	-0.1007	-0.2931	0.5684	0.4539	0.4554	-0.6211	-0.2277	-0.3456
X5	0.5564	0.6075	0.2732	0.7601	1.0000	-0.6474	-0.4119	0.7629	0.7169	0.6399	-0.7017	-0.4476	-0.5177
X6	0.0397	-0.2132	-0.1357	-0.1007	-0.6474	1.0000	0.2307	-0.4805	-0.5034	-0.3768	0.3883	0.3900	0.3478
X7	-0.2912	-0.2893	-0.0930	-0.2931	-0.4119	0.2307	1.0000	-0.5546	-0.6497	-0.4804	0.7322	0.7778	0.5236
X8	0.5697	0.6585	0.2267	0.5684	0.7629	-0.4805	-0.5546	1.0000	0.9217	0.9052	-0.6523	-0.6408	-0.6450
X9	0.5553	0.5660	0.1461	0.4539	0.7169	-0.5034	-0.6497	0.9217	1.0000	0.7883	-0.6457	-0.7173	-0.7071
X10	0.3448	0.5085	0.4195	0.4554	0.6399	-0.3768	-0.4804	0.9052	0.7883	1.0000	-0.5824	-0.6669	-0.7286
X11	-0.4672	-0.3995	-0.2235	-0.6211	-0.7017	0.3883	0.7322	-0.6523	-0.6457	-0.5824	1.0000	0.7958	0.7442
X12	-0.2496	-0.2601	-0.1776	-0.2277	-0.4476	0.3900	0.7778	-0.6408	-0.7173	-0.6669	0.7958	1.0000	0.8636
X13	-0.2711	-0.3050	-0.3803	-0.3456	-0.5177	0.3478	0.5236	-0.6450	-0.7071	-0.7286	0.7442	0.8636	1.0000

19. Results for: REV_C10_19.mtw

Correlations: C1, C2, C3, C4, C5, C6, C7, C8

	C1	C2	C3	C4	C5	C6	C7
C2	0.123						
C3	0.115	0.963					
C4	0.417	-0.063	-0.041				
C5	0.005	-0.102	-0.103	-0.059			
C6	0.001	0.270	0.295	-0.036	0.137		
C7	-0.113	-0.074	-0.076	0.052	0.134	0.061	
C8	0.077	-0.002	-0.023	0.146	0.165	-0.202	-0.032

Chapter 11

11.2.1. Results for: EXR_C11_S02_02.mtw

mobilizer: 0 G - CSF, 1 - Etoposide

With an interaction model, the interaction was not significant.
Without interaction, we obtain the following:

```
The regression equation is
conc = 12.9 - 0.0757 age - 5.48 method

Predictor        Coef     SE Coef          T        P
Constant       12.933       2.787       4.64    0.000
age          -0.07566     0.04388      -1.72    0.092
method         -5.480       1.429      -3.83    0.000

S = 3.965      R-Sq = 27.1%     R-Sq(adj) = 23.6%
```

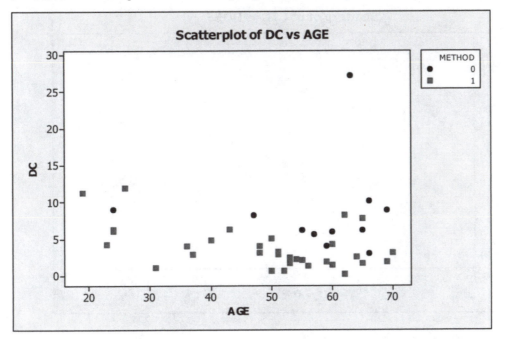

11.2.3. Results for: EXR_C11_S02_03.mtw

A model with interaction did not have interaction significant. Neither did a model containing sex. This is not surprising from the scatterplot.

Regression Analysis: QTC versus DOSE

```
The regression equation is
QTC = 560 + 0.140 DOSE


Predictor      Coef  SE Coef       T       P
Constant     559.90    29.13   19.22   0.000
DOSE        0.13989  0.06033    2.32   0.035


S = 68.2755    R-Sq = 26.4%   R-Sq(adj) = 21.5%
```

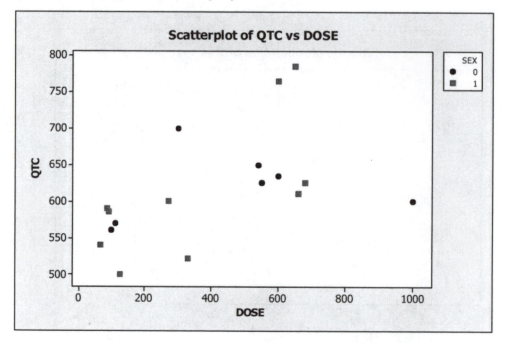

11.3.1. Results for: EXR_C11_S03_01.mtw

Stepwise Regression: MMO versus AGE, DOWNCON, ...

```
Forward selection.  Alpha-to-Enter: 0.25
```

Step	1	2	3
Constant	51.93	116.07	115.54
MEM	0.66	0.60	0.57
T-Value	5.75	5.87	5.53
P-Value	0.000	0.000	0.000
SOCIALSU		-0.476	-0.492
T-Value		-5.28	-5.51
P-Value		0.000	0.000
CGDUR			0.122
T-Value			1.88
P-Value			0.064
S	17.4	15.4	15.2
R-Sq	25.20	41.92	43.97
R-Sq(adj)	24.44	40.72	42.22

It would be up to the investigator to include CGDUR in the model since its *p* value is very close to .05. MINITAB identifies variables with *p* values at .25 or less.

11.3.3. Results for: EXR_C11_S03_03.mtw

Stepwise Regression: REACTIVE versus AGE, VERBALIQ, ...
```
Forward selection.  Alpha-to-Enter: 0.25
  Alpha-to-Enter: 0.15  Alpha-to-Remove: 0.15

Response is REACTIVE on  6 predictors, with N =    68
```

Step	1	2	3
Constant	3.374	5.476	5.418
AGEABUSE	-0.38	-0.45	-0.42
T-Value	-2.49	-3.00	-2.91
P-Value	0.015	0.004	0.005
VERBALIQ		-0.0219	-0.0228
T-Value		-2.75	-2.93
P-Value		0.008	0.005
STIM			0.61
T-Value			2.05
P-Value			0.044
S	1.06	1.01	0.990
R-Sq	8.57	18.10	23.15
R-Sq(adj)	7.19	15.58	19.55
C-p	10.4	4.6	2.5

11.4.1.

Coding sex=0 for men and sex=1 for women, vict=0 for not victimized and vict=1 for victimized, yields the following results in SAS.

```
                                Standard      Wald
        Parameter    DF  Estimate    Error   Chi-Square   Pr > ChiSq

        Intercept    1    2.1192    0.1740   148.3439      <.0001
        sex          1    0.0764    0.2159     0.1252      0.7234

                        Odds Ratio Estimates

                          Point        95% Wald
              Effect    Estimate    Confidence Limits

              sex         1.079      0.707      1.648
```

There is not a statistically significant difference with respect to gender. The odds of violent victimization are approximately equal for men and women.

Chapter 11 Review Exercises

15. Results for: REV_C11_15.mtw

Regression Analysis: CARDIAC versus VO2, DUMMY

Dummy is coded so Child = 0 and Adult = 1

```
The regression equation is
CARDIAC = 1.87 + 6.38 VO2 + 1.93 DUMMY


Predictor    Coef  SE Coef      T      P
Constant   1.8670   0.3182   5.87  0.000
VO2        6.3772   0.3972  16.06  0.000
DUMMY      1.9251   0.3387   5.68  0.000


S = 0.838601   R-Sq = 94.2%   R-Sq(adj) = 93.7%


Analysis of Variance

Source          DF     SS      MS      F      P
Regression       2  284.65  142.33  202.38  0.000
Residual Error  25   17.58    0.70
Total           27  302.23
```

17. $\hat{y} = -1.1361 + .07648x_1 + .7433x_2 - .8239x_3 - .02772x_1x_2 + .03204x_1x_3$

Coefficient	Standard deviation	t	p^a
-1.13610	.49040	-2.32	$.05 > p > .02$
.07648	.01523	5.02	$< .01$
.74330	.63880	1.16	$> .20$
-.82390	.62980	-1.31	$.20 > p > .10$
-.02772	.02039	-1.36	$.20 > p > .10$
.03204	.01974	1.62	$.20 > p > .10$

[a]Approximate. Obtained by using 35 d.f.
$R^2 = .834$

Source	SS	d.f.	MS	V.R.
Regression	3.03754	5	.60751	34.04325
Residual	.60646	34	.01784	
	3.64400	39		

$$x_2 = \begin{cases} 1 \text{ if } A \\ 0 \text{ if otherwise} \end{cases} \quad x_3 = \begin{cases} 1 \text{ if } B \\ 0 \text{ if otherwise} \end{cases}$$

For A: $\hat{y} = (-1.1361 + .7433) + (.07648 - .02772)x_1 = -.3928 + .04875x_1$

For B: $\hat{y} = (-1.1361 + .8239) + (.07648 + .03204)x_1 = -1.96 + .10852x_1$

For C: $\hat{y} = -1.1361 + .07648x_1$

23. Results for: REV_C11_23.mtw

Regression Analysis: V versus W, DUMMY1, DUMMY2, INTER1, INTER2

Response = V, Dummy1 = 1 if infant, 0 otherwise, Dummy2 = 1 if Child, 0 otherwise

```
The regression equation is
V = 11.7 + 0.137 W - 11.4 DUMMY1 - 11.7 DUMMY2 + 0.226 INTER1 + 0.223 INTER2


Predictor     Coef   SE Coef      T      P
Constant    11.750     3.822   3.07  0.004
W          0.13738   0.05107   2.69  0.010
DUMMY1     -11.421     4.336  -2.63  0.012
DUMMY2     -11.731     3.966  -2.96  0.005
INTER1      0.2264    0.2208   1.03  0.311
INTER2     0.22332   0.06714   3.33  0.002


S = 1.73234   R-Sq = 94.9%   R-Sq(adj) = 94.3%
```

Analysis of Variance

Source	DF	SS	MS	F	P
Regression	5	2304.47	460.89	153.58	0.000
Residual Error	41	123.04	3.00		
Total	46	2427.51			

Source	DF	Seq SS
W	1	2265.07
DUMMY1	1	5.59
DUMMY2	1	0.00
INTER1	1	0.60
INTER2	1	33.20

Unusual Observations

Obs	W	V	Fit	SE Fit	Residual	St Resid
17	10.8	8.366	4.257	0.496	4.109	2.48R
36	47.0	15.400	16.971	1.145	-1.571	-1.21 X
41	96.0	20.000	24.938	1.265	-4.938	-4.17RX
46	87.0	30.900	23.702	0.881	7.198	4.83R

R denotes an observation with a large standardized residual.
X denotes an observation whose X value gives it large influence.

25. Results for: REV_C11_25.mtw

Regression Analysis: IFIBRIN versus PLASMA, DUMMY1, ...

Dummy1 = 1 if drug = Endotoxin only, 0 otherwise
Dummy2 = 1 if drug = Endotoxin+PRAP-1 low dose, 0 othersise

The regression equation is
IFIBRIN = - 23.2 + 0.581 PLASMA + 74.5 DUMMY1 + 58.8 DUMMY2 + 0.025 INTER1
          - 0.263 INTER2

Predictor	Coef	SE Coef	T	P
Constant	-23.22	47.32	-0.49	0.628
PLASMA	0.5808	0.3058	1.90	0.070
DUMMY1	74.46	60.53	1.23	0.231
DUMMY2	58.78	66.52	0.88	0.386
INTER1	0.0247	0.3479	0.07	0.944
INTER2	-0.2627	0.3906	-0.67	0.508

S = 41.1074   R-Sq = 72.2%   R-Sq(adj) = 66.4%

Analysis of Variance

Source	DF	SS	MS	F	P
Regression	5	105331	21066	12.47	0.000
Residual Error	24	40556	1690		
Total	29	145887			

```
Source   DF   Seq SS
PLASMA    1   68519
DUMMY1    1   34427
DUMMY2    1     707
INTER1    1     914
INTER2    1     764
```

Unusual Observations

```
Obs  PLASMA  IFIBRIN     Fit  SE Fit  Residual  St Resid
  9     414   272.00  301.89   35.73    -29.89   -1.47 X
 13     248   187.00  114.43   20.14     72.57    2.03R
 18     276    17.00  123.33   25.72   -106.33   -3.32R
```

R denotes an observation with a large standardized residual.
X denotes an observation whose X value gives it large influence.

27. Results for: REV_C11_27.mtw

Regression Analysis: SPX versus SPNG, SIDE

Side = 0 for right side and 1 for left side

```
The regression equation is
SPX = 0.11 + 1.05 SPNG - 0.40 SIDE
```

```
Predictor     Coef  SE Coef      T      P
Constant     0.106    1.832   0.06  0.954
SPNG        1.0496   0.1268   8.28  0.000
SIDE        -0.403    1.882  -0.21  0.832
```

```
S = 5.41425   R-Sq = 69.6%   R-Sq(adj) = 67.8%
```

Analysis of Variance

```
Source           DF      SS      MS      F      P
Regression        2  2283.0  1141.5  38.94  0.000
Residual Error   34   996.7    29.3
Total            36  3279.7
```

```
Source  DF  Seq SS
SPNG     1  2281.7
SIDE     1     1.3
```

Unusual Observations

```
Obs  SPNG     SPX     Fit  SE Fit  Residual  St Resid
  5  22.0  35.900  23.196   1.904    12.704     2.51R
  7   2.3  13.600   2.520   1.630    11.080     2.15R
 15  35.9  47.700  37.785   3.438     9.915     2.37RX
```

R denotes an observation with a large standardized residual.
X denotes an observation whose X value gives it large influence.

29. Results for: REV_C11_29.mtw

<table>
<tr><td colspan="2">

Stepwise Regression: LOWESTEX versus YEARS, BMI, PAO2, PACO2, FEV

```
Alpha-to-Enter: 0.15
Alpha-to-Remove:
0.15


Response is LOWESTEX
on 5 predictors,
with N = 19



Step           1
Constant   55.31

PAO2        0.42
T-Value     4.18
P-Value     0.001

S           5.10
R-Sq       50.68
R-Sq(adj)  47.78
Mallows C-p   0.5
```

</td><td>

Stepwise Regression: MEANSLEE versus YEARS, BMI, PAO2, PACO2, FEV

```
Alpha-to-Enter: 0.15
Alpha-to-Remove:
0.15


Response is MEANSLEE
on 5 predictors,
with N = 19



Step           1
Constant   49.82

PAO2       0.541
T-Value     7.12
P-Value     0.000

S           3.88
R-Sq       74.88
R-Sq(adj)  73.40
Mallows C-p   1.3
```

</td></tr>
</table>

Stepwise Regression: LOWSLEEP versus YEARS, BMI, PAO2, PACO2, FEV

```
Alpha-to-Enter: 0.15  Alpha-to-Remove: 0.15

Response is LOWSLEEP on 5 predictors, with N =
19

Step             1       2       3       4
Constant     19.08  -18.58  -34.18  -60.53

PAO2          0.83    0.91    0.97    1.12
T-Value       6.49    6.96    7.47    7.34
P-Value      0.000   0.000   0.000   0.000

YEARS                 0.50    0.82    0.78
T-Value               1.65    2.36    2.37
P-Value              0.118   0.032   0.033

FEV                          -0.31   -0.45
T-Value                      -1.64   -2.26
P-Value                      0.122   0.040

BMI                                   0.93
T-Value                               1.65
P-Value                              0.121

S             6.57    6.26    5.96    5.64
R-Sq         71.27   75.45   79.17   82.56
R-Sq(adj)    69.58   72.38   75.01   77.58
Mallows C-p    6.6     5.4     4.6     4.1
```

Stepwise Regression: LOWSLEEP versus YEARS, BMI, PAO2, PACO2, FEV

Alpha-to-Enter: 0.15   Alpha-to-Remove: 0.15

Response is LOWSLEEP on 5 predictors, with N = 19

Step	1	2	3	4
Constant	19.08	-18.58	-34.18	-60.53
PAO2	0.83	0.91	0.97	1.12
T-Value	6.49	6.96	7.47	7.34
P-Value	0.000	0.000	0.000	0.000
YEARS		0.50	0.82	0.78
T-Value		1.65	2.36	2.37
P-Value		0.118	0.032	0.033
FEV			-0.31	-0.45
T-Value			-1.64	-2.26
P-Value			0.122	0.040
BMI				0.93
T-Value				1.65
P-Value				0.121
S	6.57	6.26	5.96	5.64
R-Sq	71.27	75.45	79.17	82.56
R-Sq(adj)	69.58	72.38	75.01	77.58
Mallows C-p	6.6	5.4	4.6	4.1

Chapter 12

12.3.1.

z	Expected relative frequency	Expected frequency	$\dfrac{(O-E)^2}{E}$
$\dfrac{1-5.74}{2.01}=-2.36$	.0091	2.275	.715
	.0223	5.575	.059
$\dfrac{2-5.74}{2.01}=-1.86$	.0555	13.875	.091
$\dfrac{3-5.74}{2.01}=-1.36$	.1053	26.325	.205
$\dfrac{4-5.74}{2.01}=-87$	.1635	40.875	.110
$\dfrac{5-5.74}{2.01}=-.37$	.1960	49.000	.020
$\dfrac{6-5.74}{2.01}=.13$	.1840	46.000	.022
$\dfrac{7-5.74}{2.01}=.63$	.1329	33.225	.313
$\dfrac{8-5.74}{2.01}=1.12$	.0788	19.700	.269
$\dfrac{9-5.74}{2.01}=1.62$	.0356	8.900	.136
$\dfrac{10-5.74}{2.01}=2.12$	.0170	4.250	.132
			2.072

$X^2 = 2.072, \text{Critical } \chi_{10}^2 = 18.307, p > .05$

12.3.3.

x	Expected relative frequency	E_i	O_i	$\dfrac{(O_i - E_i)^2}{E_i}$
0	.1074	10.74	8	.699
1	.2684	26.84	25	.126
2	.3020	30.20	32	.107
3	.2013	20.13	24	.744
4	.0881	8.81	10	.161
5	.0264	2.64 ⎫		
6	.0055	0.55 ⎪		
7	.0008	0.08 ⎬ 3.28	1	1.58
8 or more	.0001	0.01 ⎭		
		100.0		$X^2 = 3.417$

$X^2 = 3.417,\ p > .10$

12.3.5. $\hat{\lambda} = \dfrac{0 + 30 + 50 + 60 + 20 + 20 + 6}{100} = 1.86 \approx 1.9$

X	O_i	E_i	$\dfrac{(O_i - E_i)^2}{E_i}$
0	15	15.0	.000
1	30	28.4	.090
2	25	27.0	.148
3	20	17.1	.492
4	5	8.1	1.186
5	4	3.1	.261
6	1	1.0	
7	0	.2	.033
	100	100.0	2.21

$X^2 = 2.21,\ p > .10$

12.4.1.
Expected counts are printed below observed counts
Chi-Square contributions are printed below expected counts

```
          C1      C2   Total
   1      62     121    183
        62.83  120.17
        0.011   0.006

   2      18      32     50
        17.17   32.83
        0.040   0.021

Total     80     153    233
```

$$X^2 = .011 + .006 + .040 + .021 = .078, df = 1, p > .10$$

12.4.3.
Expected counts are printed below observed counts
Chi-Square contributions are printed below expected counts

```
          C1       C2    Total
   1     294      921     1215
        77.26  1137.74
       608.095  41.291

   2      98     2862     2960
       188.21  2771.79
        43.238   2.936

   3      50     3064     3114
       198.00  2916.00
       110.628   7.512

   4     203     2652     2855
       181.53  2673.47
         2.538   0.172

Total    645     9499    10144
```

Chi-Sq = 816.410, DF = 3, P-Value = 0.000

There is sufficient evidence to reject the null hypothesis.

12.4.5.
```
Expected counts are printed below observed counts
Chi-Square contributions are printed below expected counts

         C1     C2    Total
  1      31     91     122
       12.20  109.80
       28.970   3.219

  2      19     359     378
       37.80  340.20
        9.350   1.039

Total    50     450     500

Chi-Sq = 42.579, DF = 1, P-Value = 0.000
```

We have sufficient evidence to reject the null hypothesis.

12.5.1.
```
Expected counts are printed below observed counts
Chi-Square contributions are printed below expected counts

         C1     C2    Total
  1      28     35      63
       27.93  35.07
        0.000   0.000

  2      19     38      57
       25.27  31.73
        1.557   1.241

  3      41     44      85
       37.69  47.31
        0.291   0.232

  4      53     60     113
       50.10  62.90
        0.167   0.133

Total   141    177     318

Chi-Sq = 3.622, DF = 3, P-Value = 0.305
```

There is not sufficient evidence to reject the null hypothesis.

12.5.3.
```
Expected counts are printed below observed counts
Chi-Square contributions are printed below expected counts

          C1      C2    Total
   1      12      15      27
        13.02   13.98
        0.080   0.074

   2      15      14      29
        13.98   15.02
        0.074   0.069

Total     27      29      56
```

Chi-Sq = 0.297, DF = 1, P-Value = 0.586

There is not sufficient evidence to reject the null hypothesis.

12.5.5.
```
Expected counts are printed below observed counts
Chi-Square contributions are printed below expected counts

          C1      C2      C3    Total
   1     102      84      64      250
        66.50   72.00  111.50
        18.951   2.000  20.235

   2      31      60     159      250
        66.50   72.00  111.50
        18.951   2.000  20.235

Total    133     144     223      500
```

Chi-Sq = 82.373, DF = 2, P-Value = 0.000

There is sufficient evidence to reject the null hypothesis.

12.6.1.

		Total
a=8	2	A=10
b=7	3	B=10
15	5	20

Since $b = 7 > 3$ (for $A = 10$, $B = 10$, $a = 8$), $p > 2(.035)=.070$. Do not reject H_0.

12.6.3.

		Total
a=16	3	A=19
b=1	6	B=7
17	9	26

Since $b = 1$ (for $A = 19$, $B = 7$, $a = 16$), $p = 2(.002) = .004$. Reject H_0.

12.7.1.

	Survival		
	No	**Yes**	**Total**
Age 50 or older	219	157	376
Younger than 50	16	355	371
Total	235	512	747

$$\widehat{RR} = \frac{219/376}{16/371} = 13.51, \quad X^2 = \frac{747(219*355 - 157*16)^2}{(235)(512)(376)(371)} = 241.3048$$

95% CI: $13.51^{1-1.96/\sqrt{241.3048}} = 9.7, 13.51^{14.96/\sqrt{241.3048}} = 18.76$

There is statistically significant evidence that older subjects do not survive at a higher rate than younger subjects.

The 95% CI generated by SAS® is 8.30, 21.98

12.7.3. $\widehat{OR} = \frac{(36)(3396)}{(168)(370)} = 1.967$

```
Expected counts are printed below observed counts
Chi-Square contributions are printed below expected counts

            C1        C2    Total
     1      36       370      406
         20.86    385.14
         10.984    0.595

     2     168      3396     3564
        183.14   3380.86
          1.251    0.068

Total     204      3766     3970

Chi-Sq = 12.898, DF = 1, P-Value = 0.000
```

12.7.5.

$$\widehat{OR}_{MH} = \frac{\dfrac{(40)(38)}{128}+\dfrac{(75)(33)}{161}}{\dfrac{(13)(37)}{128}+\dfrac{(15)(38)}{161}} = \frac{11.875+15.373}{3.758+3.540} = 3.733$$

$$e_1 = \frac{(77)(53)}{128} = 31.883, \quad e_2 = \frac{(113)(90)}{161} = 63.168, \quad v_1 = \frac{(77)(51)(53)(75)}{128^2 127} = 7.502, \quad v_2 = \frac{(113)(48)(90)(71)}{161^2 160} = 8.3$$

$$\chi^2_{MH} = \frac{[(40+75)-(31.883+63.168)]^2}{7.502+8.357} = 25.094$$

Reject the null hypothesis, we conclude there is a relationship between garden ownership and food insecurity among employed and non-employed families.

12.8.1. SPSS for MS Windows Release 11.0.1

Survival Analysis for TIME

Time	Status	Cumulative Survival	Standard Error	Cumulative Events	Number Remaining
0	doc			0	52
1	mtc			1	51
1	mtc			2	50
1	mtc			3	49
1	mtc			4	48
1	mtc			5	47
1	mtc			6	46
1	mtc	.8654	.0473	7	45
1	alive			7	44
2	mtc			8	43
2	mtc			9	42
2	mtc	.8064	.0550	10	41
2	alive			10	40
2	alive			10	39
3	mtc			11	38
3	mtc	.7650	.0595	12	37
3	alive			12	36
4	mtc	.7438	.0615	13	35
4	alive			13	34
4	alive			13	33
4	alive			13	32
5	alive			13	31
5	alive			13	30
5	alive			13	29
5	alive			13	28
6	alive			13	27
6	alive			13	26
6	alive			13	25
6	alive			13	24
6	alive			13	23
6	alive			13	22
7	mtc	.7100	.0673	14	21
8	alive			14	20
8	alive			14	19
8	alive			14	18
8	alive			14	17
8	alive			14	16
9	alive			14	15
10	alive			14	14
11	mtc	.6593	.0794	15	13
11	doc			15	12
12	mtc	.6043	.0898	16	11
12	doc			16	10
13	mtc	.5439	.0991	17	9
14	alive			17	8
15	alive			17	7
16	mtc	.4662	.1113	18	6
16	alive			18	5
16	alive			18	4
16	alive			18	3
17	doc			18	2
18	mtc	.2331	.1740	19	1
19	alive			19	0

Number of Cases: 53   Censored: 34   (64.15%)   Events: 19

	Survival Time	Standard Error	95% Confidence Interval	
Mean:	13	1	(10,	15)
(Limited to	19)			
Median:	16	2	(12,	20)

	Percentiles		
	25.00	50.00	75.00
Value	18.00	16.00	4.00
Standard Error	.	1.80	3.76

12.8.5.

Survival Analysis for WEEKS

Factor GROUP = 1

Time	Status	Cumulative Survival	Standard Error	Cumulative Events	Number Remaining
6	G+	.9600	.0392	1	24
8	G+	.9200	.0543	2	23
14	L			2	22
16	G+	.8782	.0660	3	21
20	G+	.8364	.0749	4	20
22	L			4	19
24	L			4	18
26	L			4	17
32	G+	.7872	.0851	5	16
32	L			5	15
34	L			5	14
40	L			5	13
52	L			5	12
60	G			6	11
60	G			7	10
60	G			8	9
60	G			9	8
60	G			10	7
60	G			11	6
60	G			12	5
60	G			13	4
60	G			14	3
60	G			15	2
60	G			16	1
60	G	.0000	.0000	17	0

Number of Cases: 25   Censored: 8   (32.00%)   Events: 17

	Survival Time	Standard Error	95% Confidence Interval	
Mean:	51	4	(43,	58)
Median:	60	0	(.,	.)

```
                    Percentiles

               25.00        50.00        75.00

Value          60.00        60.00        60.00
Standard Error      .            .            .
```

Survival Analysis for WEEKS

Factor GROUP = 2

Time	Status	Cumulative Survival	Standard Error	Cumulative Events	Number Remaining
2	G+	.9600	.0392	1	24
3	G+	.9200	.0543	2	23
4	G+	.8800	.0650	3	22
6	G+	.8400	.0733	4	21
7	G+			5	20
7	G+	.7600	.0854	6	19
8	G+			7	18
8	G+	.6800	.0933	8	17
10	G+			9	16
10	G+	.6000	.0980	10	15
10	L			10	14
12	G+	.5571	.0999	11	13
15	G+	.5143	.1010	12	12
18	G+	.4714	.1013	13	11
18	L			13	10
20	G+			14	9
20	G+	.3771	.1006	15	8
22	G+			16	7
22	G+	.2829	.0950	17	6
24	G+	.2357	.0901	18	5
26	G+	.1886	.0835	19	4
27	G+	.1414	.0748	20	3
28	G+	.0943	.0630	21	2
32	G+	.0471	.0459	22	1
36	G+	.0000	.0000	23	0

```
Number of Cases:  25     Censored:   2    (  8.00%)    Events: 23

           Survival Time   Standard Error   95% Confidence Interval

Mean:          17                2         (     13,      21 )
Median:        18                5         (      9,      27 )
```

```
                    Percentiles

               25.00        50.00        75.00

Value          24.00        18.00         8.00
Standard Error  2.87         4.50         1.17
```
—

Survival Analysis for WEEKS

		Total	Number Events	Number Censored	Percent Censored
GROUP	1	25	17	8	32.00
GROUP	2	25	23	2	8.00
Overall		50	40	10	20.00

Chapter 12 Review Exercises

15.

Expected counts are printed below observed counts
Chi-Square contributions are printed below expected counts

	C1	C2	C3	C4	Total
1	611	34	16	18	679
	609.38	29.18	21.88	18.57	
	0.004	0.798	1.581	0.017	
2	308	10	17	10	345
	309.62	14.82	11.12	9.43	
	0.009	1.570	3.112	0.034	
Total	919	44	33	28	1024

Chi-Sq = 7.124, DF = 3, P-Value = 0.068

There is not sufficient evidence to reject null hypothesis.

17.

Expected counts are printed below observed counts
Chi-Square contributions are printed below expected counts

	C1	C2	Total
1	72	230	302
	69.69	232.31	
	0.076	0.023	
2	54	192	246
	56.77	189.23	
	0.135	0.041	
3	16	63	79
	18.23	60.77	
	0.273	0.082	
4	8	15	23
	5.31	17.69	
	1.366	0.410	
Total	150	500	650

Chi-Sq = 2.405, DF = 3, P-Value = 0.493

There is not sufficient evidence to reject the null hypothesis.

19.

m_i	$m_i f_i$	$m_i^2 f_i$	$z = (x_i - \overline{x})/s$
12	36	432	-2.30
17	136	2312	-1.91
22	286	6292	-1.53
27	459	12393	-1.14
32	608	19456	-.75
27	925	34225	-.26
42	1176	49392	.02
47	940	44180	.41
52	936	48672	.80
57	684	38988	1.18
62	496	30752	1.57
67	268	17956	1.96
	6950	305050	

Expected relative frequency	Expected frequency	$\dfrac{(O_i - E_i)^2}{E_i}$
.0107	1.872	1.8720
.0174	3.045	.0007
.0349	6.108	.5861
.0641	11.218	.2831
.0995	17.412	.0097
.1328	23.240	.7736
.1486	26.005	.0388
.1511	26.442	.0918
.1290	22.575	.2937
.0929	16.258	.1866
.0608	10.640	.1738
.0332	5.810	.8255
.0250	4.375	.0321
		$X^2 = 5.1675$

$$\overline{x} = 6950/175 = 39.71, \quad s^2 = \frac{175(305,050) - (6950)^2}{(175)(174)} = 166.8719$$

$s = 12.92, \quad p > .10$ Do not reject H_0.

21.

```
Expected counts are printed below observed counts
Chi-Square contributions are printed below expected counts

          C1      C2      C3   Total
     1    80     100      20     200
        71.65   92.09   36.26
        0.972   0.680   7.291

     2    99     190      96     385
       137.94  177.27   69.80
       10.990   0.915   9.836

     3    70      30      10     110
        39.41   50.65   19.94
       23.744   8.417   4.957

Total   249     320     126     695

Chi-Sq = 67.802, DF = 4, P-Value = 0.000
```

There is sufficient evidence to reject the null hypothesis.

23.

```
Expected counts are printed below observed counts
Chi-Square contributions are printed below expected counts

          C1      C2   Total
     1   111     102     213
        96.82  116.18
        2.077   1.731

     2    59      73     132
        60.00   72.00
        0.017   0.014

     3    80     125     205
        93.18  111.82
        1.865   1.554

Total   250     300     550

Chi-Sq = 7.258, DF = 2, P-Value = 0.027
```

There is sufficient evidence to reject the null hypothesis, $.025 < p < .05$.

29.

Variables: Treatment (2 levels of imiquimod-treated and control cream) and Result (two levels of success and failure). These are qualitative variables. The null hypothesis is the proportion of success is the same with the imiquimod cream as the control cream. The alternative is that the proportion of success is not the same with the two creams. The conclusion is to reject the null hypothesis.

33. This is a retrospective study. The variables are qualitative with the risk factor of living in area of high road traffic exhaust and a response variable as childhood leukemia. The children living in the high exhaust areas had odds almost 4 times higher for contracting childhood leukemia than comparable children in non-traffic exhaust areas.

35. Satisfaction
Expected counts are printed below observed counts
Chi-Square contributions are printed below expected counts

```
         UH      MH      HD   Total
  1       5       9       6      20
         7.00    9.00    4.00
         0.571   0.000   1.000

  2       9       9       2      20
         7.00    9.00    4.00
         0.571   0.000   1.000

Total    14      18       8      40
```

Chi-Sq = 3.143, DF = 2, P-Value = 0.208
2 cells with expected counts less than 5.

Pain
Expected counts are printed below observed counts
Chi-Square contributions are printed below expected counts

```
         UH      MH      HD   Total
  1       2      10       8      20
         2.00    9.00    9.00
         0.000   0.111   0.111

  2       2       8      10      20
         2.00    9.00    9.00
         0.000   0.111   0.111

Total     4      18      18      40
```

Chi-Sq = 0.444, DF = 2, P-Value = 0.801
2 cells with expected counts less than 5.

Nausea
Expected counts are printed below observed counts
Chi-Square contributions are printed below expected counts

```
         UB      MO      SL   Total
  1       5       9       6      20
         6.00    8.50    5.50
         0.167   0.029   0.045

  2       7       8       5      20
         6.00    8.50    5.50
         0.167   0.029   0.045

Total    12      17      11      40
```

Chi-Sq = 0.483, DF = 2, P-Value = 0.785

37.

	M	**F**	**Total**
W	29	9	38
$\bar{W}$	94	60	154
Total	123	69	192

$$\widehat{OR} = \frac{(29)(60)}{(9)(94)} = 2.06, \quad X^2 = \frac{192(1740 - 846)^2}{(123)(69)(154)(38)} = 3.0897$$

95% CI: $2.06^{1-1.96/\sqrt{3.0897}} = .92,\ 2.06^{14.96/\sqrt{3.0897}} = 4.61$

41.
```
Expected counts are printed below observed counts
Chi-Square contributions are printed below expected counts

          M      F   Total
    1    47      6      53
       37.98  15.02
       2.140  5.414

    2    39     28      67
       48.02  18.98
       1.693  4.283

Total    86     34     120

Chi-Sq = 13.530, DF = 1, P-Value = 0.000
```

43. Fisher's Exact Test

Post Operative Complication	Ultrasonic Appearance of Fetal Bowel		Total
	Normal	**Not Normal**	
No	13	5	18
Yes	2	7	9
Total	15	12	27

Test statistic = 2, $p = .019$

45.

```
Expected counts are printed below observed counts
Chi-Square contributions are printed below expected counts

        40-69      >=70   Total
   1       21        17      38
        28.79      9.21
        2.106      6.580

   2     4000      1270    5270
      3992.21   1277.79
        0.015      0.047

Total   4021      1287    5308

Chi-Sq = 8.749, DF = 1, P-Value = 0.003
```

47.

```
Expected counts are printed below observed counts
Chi-Square contributions are printed below expected counts

        Cures   Failures   Total
   1       22         10      32
        17.26      14.74
        1.300      1.523

   2       19         25      44
        23.74      20.26
        0.945      1.107

Total      41         35      76

Chi-Sq = 4.875, DF = 1, P-Value = 0.027
```

49.

Smoker	HPV+	HPV-	Total
Yes	44	6	50
No	60	31	91
Total	104	37	141

$$\widehat{OR} = \frac{44/6}{60/31} = 3.79, \quad X^2 = 8.1178, \quad 95\% \text{ CI } 3.79^{1+.96/\sqrt{8.1178}} = 1.52, \quad 3.79^{1+.96/\sqrt{8.1178}} = 9.48$$

SAS® 95% CI 1.46, 9.86

51. Expected counts are printed below observed counts
Chi-Square contributions are printed below expected counts

	SC	IV	Total
1	11	24	35
	17.50	17.50	
	2.414	2.414	
2	19	6	25
	12.50	12.50	
	3.380	3.380	

Total   30   30   60
Chi-Sq = 11.589, DF = 1, P-Value = 0.001

53. Survival Analysis for MONTHS

Factor NUMBER = >1

Time	Status	Cumulative Survival	Standard Error	Cumulative Events	Number Remaining
.000000	D	.9677	.0317	1	30
3.000000	D	.9355	.0441	2	29
7.000000	D			3	28
7.000000	D	.8710	.0602	4	27
8.000000	D	.8387	.0661	5	26
9.000000	D	.8065	.0710	6	25
10.00000	D			7	24
10.00000	D	.7419	.0786	8	23
15.00000	D			9	22
15.00000	D	.6774	.0840	10	21
16.00000	D	.6452	.0859	11	20
17.00000	D	.6129	.0875	12	19
18.00000	D	.5806	.0886	13	18
20.00000	D			14	17
20.00000	D	.5161	.0898	15	16
23.00000	D	.4839	.0898	16	15
24.00000	D	.4516	.0894	17	14
26.00000	D	.4194	.0886	18	13
27.00000	D	.3871	.0875	19	12
28.00000	D	.3548	.0859	20	11
29.00000	D	.3226	.0840	21	10
30.00000	D	.2903	.0815	22	9
33.00000	D	.2581	.0786	23	8
41.00000	D			24	7
41.00000	D	.1935	.0710	25	6
42.00000	A			25	5
57.00000	A			25	4
73.00000	A			25	3
73.00000	A			25	2
99.00000	D	.0968	.0771	26	1
129.0000	A			26	0

Number of Cases: 31   Censored: 5   (16.13%)   Events: 26

	Survival Time	Standard Error	95% Confidence Interval
Mean:	37.451613	7.256392	(23.229084, 51.674142)
(Limited to	129.00)		
Median:	23.000000	4.451893	(14.274289, 31.725711)

Survival Analysis for MONTHS
Factor NUMBER = 1

Time	Status	Cumulative Survival	Standard Error	Cumulative Events	Number Remaining
2.000000	D	.9783	.0215	1	45
3.000000	A			1	44
5.000000	D	.9560	.0304	2	43
10.00000	D			3	42
10.00000	D	.9116	.0422	4	41
14.00000	D	.8893	.0467	5	40
15.00000	D			6	39
15.00000	D	.8449	.0539	7	38
16.00000	D	.8226	.0569	8	37
17.00000	D			9	36
17.00000	D	.7782	.0619	10	35
18.00000	D	.7559	.0640	11	34
19.00000	D	.7337	.0659	12	33
19.00000	A			12	32
24.00000	A			12	31
24.00000	A			12	30
26.00000	D			13	29
26.00000	D	.6848	.0700	14	28
27.00000	D			15	27
27.00000	D	.6359	.0730	16	26
29.00000	D	.6114	.0742	17	25
29.00000	A			17	24
33.00000	D	.5859	.0753	18	23
35.00000	A			18	22
37.00000	D	.5593	.0765	19	21
39.00000	A			19	20
40.00000	A			19	19
41.00000	D	.5299	.0779	20	18
42.00000	A			20	17
43.00000	D			21	16
43.00000	D	.4675	.0803	22	15
45.00000	A			22	14
46.00000	D	.4341	.0812	23	13
54.00000	D	.4007	.0815	24	12
55.00000	A			24	11
60.00000	D	.3643	.0818	25	10
66.00000	A			25	9
67.00000	A			25	8
74.00000	A			25	7
92.00000	A			25	6
93.00000	A			25	5
121.0000	A			25	4
127.0000	A			25	3
133.0000	A			25	2
143.0000	A			25	1
169.0000	A			25	0

Number of Cases: 46   Censored: 21   (45.65%)   Events: 25

	Survival Time	Standard Error	95% Confidence Interval
Mean:	79.620583	11.336661	(57.400728, 101.84044)
(Limited to 169.00)			
Median:	43.000000	5.770779	(31.689272, 54.310728)

—   ʼ

Survival Analysis for MONTHS

		Total	Number Events	Number Censored	Percent Censored
NUMBER	>1	31	26	5	16.13
NUMBER	1	46	25	21	45.65
Overall		77	51	26	33.77

Chapter 13

13.3.1. H_0: median = 100, H_A: median $\neq 100$

Sign of x $-$ 100: -, -, -, +, +, -, +, -, -, +, -, +, +, -, -

$P(k \leq 6 | 15, .5) = .3036$, $p = 2(.3036) = .6072$, fail to reject the null hypothesis.

13.3.3.

Subj	1	2	3	4	5	6	7	8	9	10	11	12	13	14	15
B-A	0	+	-	-	0	-	-	-	+	-	-	-	-	-	-

$P(x \leq 2 | 13, .5) = .0112$, reject the null hypothesis

13.4.1.

$d_i = x_i - 70$	Signed Rank of d_i
-7	-14.5
-2	-2
9	16
-5	-8.5
-6	-11.5
-7	-14.5
-5	-8.5
-6	-11.5
6	11.5
4	6
-4	-6
-4	-6
-3	-3.5
3	3.5
-1	-1
6	11.5

$T_+ = 48.5$ $T_- = 87.5$ Since $48.5 > 36$, cannot reject the null hypothesis.

Since $48 < 48.5 < 49$, we have $.1613 < p < .1742$

13.4.3.

	LVEDV (mL)			
Subject	Baseline	5 Minutes	Diff	Rank
1	51.7	49.3	2.4	1
2	79.0	72.0	7.0	2
3	78.7	87.3	-8.6	-4
4	80.3	88.3	-8.0	-3
5	72.0	103.3	-31.3	-10
6	85.0	94.0	-9.0	-5
7	69.7	94.7	-25.0	-8.5
8	71.3	46.3	25.0	8.5
9	55.7	71.7	-16.0	-6.5
10	56.3	72.3	-16.0	-6.5

$T_+ = 43.5$ $\qquad$ $T_- = 11.5$

$T = 11.5$, $2(.0527) < p < 2(.0654)$ which implies $.1054 < p < .1308$ MINITAB p value $.114$

Fail to reject the null hypothesis.

13.5.1. Median $= 79.5$

	Hospital		
	A	B	Total
Above Median	13	2	15
Below Median	2	13	15
Total	15	15	30

$$X^2 = \frac{30(13*13-2*2)^2}{(15)(15)(15)(15)} = 16.13333 \quad \text{Since } 16.13333 > 3.841, \text{ reject the null hypothesis, } p < .005$$

13.6.1. Sum of the ranks for group 1 is 1378.5 and for group 2 it is 1106.5. Let $S = 1378.5$ and thus $T = 1378.5 - \dfrac{34(35)}{2} = 712.5$. Since both groups have sample sizes greater than 20, we use

$z = \dfrac{712.5 - [(36)(34)/2]}{\sqrt{36(34)(36+34+1)/12}} = 1.18$, which yields a two sided p value of $.1190(2) = .2380$. We fail to reject H_0.

13.6.3. Sum of the ranks for group 1 is 1772.50 and for group 2 it is 1713.5. Let $S = 1772.50$ and

thus $T = 1772.5 - \dfrac{43(44)}{2} = 826.5$. Since both groups have sample sizes greater than 20, we use

$z = \dfrac{826.5 - [(43)(40)/2]}{\sqrt{43(40)(43+40+1)/12}} = -.31$. The 2-sided p value is $2(.3783) = .7566$. Fail to reject H_0.

13.7.1.

x	$z = (x-1050)/50$	$F_T(x)$	Freq
859	-3.82	0.0001	1
904	-2.92	0.0018	1
920	-2.60	0.0047	1
962	-1.76	0.0392	1
973	-1.54	0.0618	1
1001	-0.98	0.1635	1
1002	-0.96	0.1695	1
1012	-0.76	0.2236	1
1016	-0.68	0.2483	1
1039	-0.22	0.4192	1
1041	-0.18	0.4286	1
1051	0.02	0.5080	1
1064	0.28	0.6103	1
1073	0.46	0.6772	1
1086	0.72	0.7642	1
1117	1.34	0.9099	1
1140	1.80	0.9641	1
1141	1.82	0.9656	1
1146	1.92	0.9726	1
1166	2.32	0.9898	1
1168	2.36	0.9909	1
1202	3.04	0.9988	1
1233	3.66	$\cong 1.0000$	1
1255	4.10	$\cong 1.0000$	1
1348	5.96	$\cong 1.0000$	1
			25

Cumulative frequency	$F_S(x)$	$\lvert F_S(x_i) - F_T(x_i) \rvert$	$\lvert F_S(x_{i-1}) - F_T(x_i) \rvert$
1	0.04	0.0400	0.0000
2	0.08	0.0782	0.0382
3	0.12	0.1153	0.0753
4	0.16	0.1208	0.0808
5	0.20	0.1382	0.0982
6	0.24	0.0765	0.0365
7	0.28	0.1115	0.0715
8	0.32	0.0964	0.0564
9	0.36	0.1117	0.0717
10	0.40	0.0192	0.0592
11	0.44	0.0114	0.0286
12	0.48	0.0280	0.0680
13	0.52	0.0903	0.1303
14	0.56	0.1172	0.1572
15	0.60	0.1642	0.2042
16	0.64	0.2699	0.3099
17	0.68	0.2841	0.3241
18	0.72	0.2456	0.2856
19	0.76	0.2126	0.2526
20	0.80	0.1898	0.2298
21	0.84	0.1509	0.1909
22	0.88	0.1188	0.1588
23	0.92	0.0800	0.1200
24	0.96	0.0400	0.0800
25	1.00	0.0000	0.0400

$D = .3241$, reject H_0. $p < .01$

13.7.3.

x	Frequency	Cumulative frequency	$F_S(x)$	$z = (x-150)/12$
130	1	1	0.05	-1.67
134	1	2	0.10	-1.33
137	1	3	0.15	-1.08
141	2	5	0.25	-0.75
143	1	6	0.30	-0.58
146	1	7	0.35	-0.33
147	1	8	0.40	-0.25
151	2	10	0.50	0.08
153	1	11	0.55	0.25
154	1	12	0.60	0.33
157	3	15	0.75	0.58
161	1	16	0.80	0.92
162	1	17	0.85	1.00
167	1	18	0.90	1.42
177	1	19	0.95	2.25
179	1	20	1.00	2.42
	20			

$F_T(x)$	$\left|F_S(x_i) - F_T(x_i)\right|$	$\left|F_S(x_{i-1}) - F_T(x_i)\right|$
0.0475	0.0025	0.0475
0.0918	0.0082	0.0418
0.1401	0.0099	0.0401
0.2266	0.0234	0.0766
0.2810	0.0190	0.0310
0.3707	0.0207	0.0707
0.4013	0.0013	0.0513
0.5319	0.0319	0.1319
0.5987	0.0487	0.0987
0.6293	0.0293	0.0793
0.7190	0.0310	0.1190
0.8212	0.0212	0.0712
0.8413	0.0087	0.0413
0.9222	0.0222	0.0722
0.9878	0.0378	0.0878
0.9922	0.0078	0.0422

$D = .1319$ Do not reject H_0. $p > .20$

13.8.1. Results for: EXR_C13_S08_01.mtw

Kruskal-Wallis Test: B12 versus GROUP

```
Kruskal-Wallis Test on B12

GROUP       N   Median  Ave Rank      Z
1          50    334.5     133.0   1.96
2          92    345.0     125.5   1.65
3          90    262.0      98.2  -3.31
Overall   232              116.5

H = 11.38   DF = 2   P = 0.003
H = 11.38   DF = 2   P = 0.003   (adjusted for ties)
```

Reject H_0.

13.8.3. Results for: EXR_C13_S08_03.mtw

Kruskal-Wallis Test: IMP versus GROUP

```
Kruskal-Wallis Test on IMP

GROUP      N   Median  Ave Rank      Z
1         23    4.000      17.1  -4.09
2          7   15.000      28.6   0.29
3         23   18.000      36.4   3.89
Overall   53               27.0

H = 18.13   DF = 2   P = 0.000
H = 18.21   DF = 2   P = 0.000   (adjusted for ties)
```

Reject H_0.

13.8.5. Results for: EXR_C13_S08_05.mtw

Kruskal-Wallis Test: PEST versus GROUP

```
Kruskal-Wallis Test on PEST

GROUP      N   Median  Ave Rank      Z
A         11   15.000      31.6   2.71
B         11   18.000      28.6   1.83
C         11   10.000      20.2  -0.68
D         11    5.000       9.5  -3.86
Overall   44               22.5

H = 19.55   DF = 3   P = 0.000
H = 19.61   DF = 3   P = 0.000   (adjusted for ties)
```

Reject H_0.

13.9.1

3	2	1
3	1	2
1	2	3
3	1	2
3	1	2
3	1	2
2	1	3
2	1	3
3	1	2
23	11	20

$$X_R^2 = \frac{12}{9(3)(3+1)}\left[23^2 + 11^2 + 20^2\right] - 3(9)(3+1) = 8.67$$

$p = .01$, Reject H_0.

Results for: EXR_C13_S09_01.mtw

Friedman Test: RESP versus AREA blocked by SUBJ

```
S = 8.67  DF = 2  P = 0.013

                    Sum
                     of
AREA  N  Est Median  Ranks
1     9     88.000   23.0
2     9     80.000   11.0
3     9     85.000   20.0

Grand median = 84.333
```

13.9.3.

SUBJ	SALINE	2	10	20	40
1	1	2.5	5	4	2.5
2	1	2	3	4	5
3	1	3	4	5	2
4	1	2	4	3	5
5	1	2	4	5	3
6	1	2	3	5	4
7	1	2	3	5	4
8	1	2	3	5	4
9	1	4	3	5	2
10	1	3	4	5	2
	10	24.5	36	46	33.5

$$X_r^2 = \frac{12}{10(5)(6)}\left[10^2 + 24.5^2 + 36^2 + 46^2 + 33.5^2\right] - 3(10)(6) = 29.38.$$ Since $29.38 > 9.488$, reject H_0. Since $29.38 > 14.860$, $p < .005$.

Friedman Test: RESP versus TREAT blocked by SUBJ

```
S = 29.38  DF = 4  P = 0.000
S = 29.53  DF = 4  P = 0.000 (adjusted for ties)

                      Sum
                       of
TREAT   N  Est Median  Ranks
SAL    10    -0.9815   10.0
T10    10    -0.2365   36.0
T2     10    -0.3395   24.5
T20    10    -0.1135   46.0
T40    10    -0.2865   33.5

Grand median = -0.3915
```

13.10.1.

d_i	d_i^2
-2	4
-12	144
8	64
-11	121
-2	4
2	4
-2	4
-2	4
-2	4
9	81
1	1
-1	1
4	16
12	144
-2	4
	600

$$r_S = 1 - \frac{6(600)}{15(15^2 - 1)} = -.07, \ p > .20.$$

Do not reject H_0.

13.10.3.

d_i	d_i^2
.00	.00
5.00	25.00
17.00	289.00
12.00	144.00
12.00	144.00
-1.00	1.00
2.00	4.00
6.00	36.00
7.50	56.25
-7.00	49.00
-4.00	16.00
-10.00	100.00
-2.50	6.25
-1.50	2.25
2.50	6.25
-4.00	16.00
.00	.00
-12.50	156.25
-8.50	72.25
-13.00	169.00
	1292.5

$$r_S = 1 - \frac{6(1292.5)}{20(20^2 - 1)} = .028, \quad p > .20$$

With MINITAB using the ranked data, the result is $r_s = .018$, $p = .939$.

Do not reject H_0.

13.10.5.

d_i	d_i^2
21.0	441.00
-5.0	25.00
27.0	729.00
-6.0	36.00
-5.0	25.00
3.0	9.00
-9.0	81.00
-13.0	169.00
-9.0	81.00
-7.0	49.00
-1.0	1.00
-5.0	25.00
17.0	289.00
16.0	256.00
-8.0	64.00
-1.0	1.00
7.5	56.25
10.0	100.00
-13.0	169.00
9.0	81.00
21.0	441.00
12.0	144.00
24.5	600.25
-26.0	676.00
-29.0	841.00
-2.0	4.00
-9.0	81.00
16.0	256.00
-23.0	529.00
-13.0	169.00
	6428.5

$$r_S = 1 - \frac{6(6428.5)}{30(30^2 - 1)} = -.43, \ .005(2) < p < .01(2) \ \text{implies} \ .01 < p < .02.$$

Reject H_0.

13.11.1. S_{ij} values

(57.4 - 53.9)	/(164 -163)	=	3.5000
(41.0 - 53.9)	/(156 - 163)	=	1.8429
(40.0 -53.9)	/(151 - 163)	=	1.1583
(42.0 - 53.9)	/(152 - 163)	=	1.0818
(64.4 - 53.9)	/(167 - 163)	=	2.6250
(59.1 - 53.9)	/(165 - 163)	=	2.6000
(49.9 - 53.9)	/(153 - 163)	=	0.4000
(43.2 - 53.9)	/(155 - 163)	=	1.3375
(41.0 -. 57.4)	/(156 - 154)	=	2.0500
(40.0 - 57.4)	/(151 - 164)	=	1.3385
(42.0 - 57.4)	/(152 - 164)	=	1.2833
(64.4 - 57.4)	/(167 - 164)	=	2.3333
(59.1 - 57.4)	/(165 - 164)	=	1.7000
(49.9 - 57.4)	/(153 - 164)	=	0.6818
(43.2 - 57.4)	/(155 - 164)	=	1.5778
(40.0 - 41.0)	/(151 - 156)	=	0.2000
(42.0 - 41.0)	/(152 - 156)	=	-0.2500
(64.4 - 41.0)	/(167 - 156)	=	2.1273
(59.1 - 41.0)	/(165 - 156)	=	2.0111
(49.9 - 41.0)	/(153 - 156)	=	-2.9667
(43.2 - 41.0)	/(155 - 156)	=	-2.2000
(42.0 - 40.0)	/(152 - 151)	=	2.0000
(64.4 - 40.0)	/(167 - 151)	=	1.5250
(59.1 - 40.0)	/(165 - 151)	=	1.3643
(49.9 - 40.0)	/(153 - 151)	=	4.9500
(43.2 - 40.0)	/(155 - 151)	=	0.8000
(64.4 - 42.0)	/(167 - 152)	=	1.4933
(59.1 - 42.0)	/(165 - 152)	=	1.3154
(49.9 - 42.0)	/(153 - 152)	=	7.9000
(43.2 - 42.0)	/(155 - 152)	=	0.4000
(59.9 - 64.4)	/(165 - 167)	=	2.6500
(49.1 - 64.4)	/(153 - 167)	=	1.0357
(43.2 - 64.4)	/(155 - 167)	=	1.7667
(49.9 - 59.1)	/(153 - 165)	=	0.7667
(43.2 - 59.1)	/(155 - 165)	=	1.5900
(43.2 - 49.9)	/(155 - 153)	=	-3.3500

$\widehat{\beta}$ = median $\{S_{ij}\}$ = 1.429

$y_i - \hat{\beta}x_i$ values:

53.9	-1.429(163) =	-179.027
57.4	-1.429(164) =	-176.956
41.0	-1.429(156) =	-181.924
40.0	-1.429(151) =	-175.779
42.0	-1.429(152) =	-175.208
64.4	-1.429(167) =	-174.243
59.1	-1.429(155) =	-176.685
49.9	-1.429(153) =	-168.737
43.2	-1.429(155) =	-178.295

$\hat{\alpha}_{1,M} = -176.685$

Ordered Pairwise averages of the $y_i - 1.429x_i$ values:

-168.737 -171.490 -171.973 -172.258 -172.711 -172.846 -173.516
-173.882 -174.243 -174.725 -175.011 -175.208 -175.331 -175.464
-175.493 -175.600 -175.779 -175.947 -176.082 -176.232 -176.269
-176.367 -176.635 -176.685 -176.751 -176.820 -176.956 -177.037
-177.117 -177.403 -177.490 -177.626 -177.856 -177.992 -178.083
-178.295 -178.566 -178.661 -178.852 -179.027 -179.305 -179.440
-180.109 -180.475 -181.924

$\hat{\alpha}_{2,M} = -176.63$

(888 — 781.7) / (706.0 — 660.2) 2.3210

Chapter 13 Review Exercises

7. All differences are greater than 0, thus $T = 0$, $n = 7$, $p = .0078$.

9.
Friedman Test: FEV versus TREAT blocked by SUBJ

```
S = 16.20  DF = 2  P = 0.000

                          Sum
                           of
TREAT   N  Est Median   Ranks
A       10     0.0333    11.0
B       10     0.1867    20.0
C       10     0.2750    29.0

Grand median = 0.1650
```

11. H_0: The population is normally distributed with $\mu = 44$ and $\sigma = 12$

H_A: The population is normally distributed with $\mu = 44$ and $\sigma = 12$

X	Frequency	Cumulative Frequency	$F_S(x)$	$z = (x - 44)/12$
32	2	2	.1250	-1.00
33	2	4	.2500	-.92
36	1	5	.3125	-.67
37	1	6	.3750	-.58
39	1	7	.4375	-.42
40	1	8	.5000	-.33
42	1	9	.5625	-.17
45	1	10	.6250	.08
48	2	12	.7500	.33
49	1	13	.8125	.42
56	1	14	.8750	1.00
60	1	15	.9375	1.33
75	1	16	1.0000	2.58

$F_T(x)$	$\left|F_S(x_i)-F_T(x_i)\right|$	$\left|F_S(x_i-1)-F_T(x_i)\right|$
.1587	.0337	.1587
.1788	.0712	.0538
.2514	.0611	.0014
.2810	.0940	.0315
.3372	.1003	.0378
.3707	.1293	.0668
.4325	.1300	.0675
.5319	.0931	.0306
.6293	.1207	.0043
.6628	.1497	.0872
.8413	.1337	.0288
.9082	.0293	.0332
.9951	.0049	.0576

$D = .1587$. Since $.1587 < .258$, cannot reject H_0. The population may be normally distributed. $p > .20$.

13. The sum of the $d_i^2 = 51989.5$ and $n = 70$. $r_S = 1 - \dfrac{6(51989.5)}{70(70^2-1)} = .09$

$z = .75, p = .2266(2) = .4532$

MINITAB correlation is $0.064, p = 0.597$

15. Results for: REV_C13_15.mtw

Mann-Whitney Test and CI: CONTROLS, PREV

```
           N   Median
CONTROLS  11    40.00
PREV      12    48.13


Point estimate for ETA1-ETA2 is -10.00
95.5 Percent CI for ETA1-ETA2 is (-17.50,-1.25)
W = 95.5
Test of ETA1 = ETA2 vs ETA1 not = ETA2 is significant at 0.0267
The test is significant at 0.0263 (adjusted for ties)
```

17. Results for: REV_C13_17.mtw

Kruskal-Wallis Test: PERC versus GROUPS

```
Kruskal-Wallis Test on PERC

GROUPS    N  Median  Ave Rank      Z
AR       32  4.5000      40.1   2.44
HT       10  4.0000      32.3  -0.31
LT       15  2.0000      32.0  -0.44
NO       10  0.5000      19.3  -2.59
Overall  67             34.0

H = 9.02  DF = 3  P = 0.029
H = 9.30  DF = 3  P = 0.026  (adjusted for ties)
```

19. Results for: REV_C13_19.mtw

Correlations: C3, C4

```
Pearson correlation of C3 and C4 = -0.036
P-Value = 0.802
```

21. Mann-Whitney Test and CI: T41, T42

```
      N  Median
T41   9   50.00
T42  34   81.50


Point estimate for ETA1-ETA2 is -34.00
95.3 Percent CI for ETA1-ETA2 is (-64.00,-8.99)
W = 107.5
Test of ETA1 = ETA2 vs ETA1 not = ETA2 is significant at 0.0072
The test is significant at 0.0072 (adjusted for ties)
```

23. USO patients only, Friedman Test: TC0USO versus TIME blocked by SUSO

```
S = 3.94  DF = 2  P = 0.140

                           Sum
                            of
TIME   N   Est Median    Ranks
0      31      168.67     53.0
2      31      178.33     66.0
4      31      179.00     67.0

Grand median = 175.33
```

BSO patients only, Friedman Test: TC versus Time blocked by SUBJ

```
S = 4.77  DF = 2  P = 0.092

                           Sum
                            of
Time   N   Est Median    Ranks
0      13      202.00     20.0
2      13      219.33     31.0
4      13      221.67     27.0

Grand median = 214.33
```

25. Let C4 = Week10 - Week0 for 60% group, Let C5 = Week10-Week0 for 10% group

Mann-Whitney Test and CI: C4, C5

```
       N  Median
C4    10   219.5
C5    10   -43.0


Point estimate for ETA1-ETA2 is 240.0
95.5 Percent CI for ETA1-ETA2 is (108.9,377.9)
W = 143.0
Test of ETA1 = ETA2 vs ETA1 not = ETA2 is significant at 0.0046
```

27. Mann-Whitney Test and CI: PFKC, PFKCOPD

```
          N  Median
PFKC      9   51.60
PFKCOPD   9   61.30


Point estimate for ETA1-ETA2 is -1.60
95.8 Percent CI for ETA1-ETA2 is (-33.58,38.29)
W = 83.0
Test of ETA1 = ETA2 vs ETA1 not = ETA2 is significant at 0.8598
```

Mann-Whitney Test and CI: HKC, HKCOPD

```
         N  Median
HKC      9   2.400
HKCOPD   9   1.600
```

```
Point estimate for ETA1-ETA2 is 0.800
95.8 Percent CI for ETA1-ETA2 is (-0.100,1.201)
W = 106.5
Test of ETA1 = ETA2 vs ETA1 not = ETA2 is significant at 0.0703
The test is significant at 0.0695 (adjusted for ties)
```

Mann-Whitney Test and CI: LDHC, LDHCOPD

```
          N  Median
LDHC      9   216.8
LDHCOPD   9   204.7
```

```
Point estimate for ETA1-ETA2 is -6.5
95.8 Percent CI for ETA1-ETA2 is (-142.2,92.3)
W = 82.0
Test of ETA1 = ETA2 vs ETA1 not = ETA2 is significant at 0.7911
```

29.

IL6	CRP	RANKIL6	RANKCRP
122	32	5.0	10.0
203	39	7.0	11.0
458	63	16.0	17.0
78	7	3.0	1.0
239	62	11.0	16.0
165	22	6.0	6.0
467	53	17.0	15.0
421	29	14.5	8.0
421	44	14.5	13.0
227	24	10.0	7.0
265	31	12.0	9.0
97	12	4.0	3.5
215	50	9.0	14.0
415	41	13.0	12.0
66	12	2.0	3.5
58	14	1.0	5.0
213	9	8.0	2.0

Correlations: RANKIL6, RANKCRP

```
Pearson correlation of RANKIL6 and RANKCRP = 0.733
P-Value = 0.001
```

Chapter 14

14.2.1. **(a)** $\dfrac{1366}{236517} * 1000 = 5.8$

(b) White: $\dfrac{898}{89741} * 1000 = 10.0$, Black: $\dfrac{446}{121927} * 1000 = 3.7$

(c) $\dfrac{41}{4350} * 1000 = 9.43$ **(d)** $\dfrac{24}{4350} * 1000 = 5.5$ **(e)** $\dfrac{41}{4350} * 1000 = 9.43$

(f) MN $\dfrac{303}{1366} * 100 = 22.2$, MCD $\dfrac{471}{1366} * 100 = 34.5$

14.2.3

Age (years)	Population[a]	Deaths[b]	U.S. Population[c]	Age-Specific death rates (per 100,000)	Standard population based on U.S. population 2000	Number of expected deaths in standard population
0-4	539,509	1,178	19,175,798	218.3	68139	149
5-14	1,113,920	224	41,077,577	20.1	145964	29
15-24	1,117,439	954	39,183,891	85.4	139235	119
25-34	1,213,415	1,384	39,891,724	114.1	141751	162
35-44	1,287,120	2,823	45,148,527	219.3	160430	352
45-54	1,085,150	5,271	37,677,952	485.7	133884	650
55-64	723,712	8,035	24,274,684	1110.2	86257	958
65 and Over	969,048	51,863	34,991,753	5352.0	124339	6655
Total	8,049,313	71,732	281,421,906	891.2	1000000	9073

Age-Adjusted death rate $= \dfrac{9073}{1,000,000} * 1000 = 9.1$

14.3.1.

Age of woman (years)	Number of women in population[a]	Number of births to women of specified age[b]	Age adusted fertility	Fertility rate	Cumulative fertility rate	Standard US population	Expected births
10-14	307,496	391	1.3	6.35780628	6.3	112,524	143.0811588
15-19	287,916	17249	59.9	299.5491741	305.9	110,835	6640.106541
20-24	294,360	37,286	126.7	633.3401277	939.2	103,951	13167.26792
25-29	309,759	34,884	112.6	563.0829128	1502.3	106,239	11964.27312
30-34	339,018	28,334	83.6	417.8834162	1920.2	112,438	9397.195111
35-39	353,387	12,911	36.5	182.6750843	2102.9	124,466	4547.367407
40-54	923,315	2,413	2.6	39.20113937	2142.1	329,546	861.2385784
Total	2,815,251	98,584	35.0	2142.089661		1,000,000	46720.52984

(a) (10-14): 1.3, (15-19): 59.9, (20-24): 126.7, (25-29): 112.6, (30-34): 83.6, (35-39): 36.5, (40-over):2.6;

(b) 2142.1

(c) (10-14): 6.3, (15-19):305.9, (20-24): 939.2, (25-29): 1502.3, (30-34): 1920.2, (35-39): 2102.9, (40-over):2142.1

(d) 46.7

14.3.3.

Age	No. of births	No. of women in population	Total	Fertility rate	Total fertility rate	Cumulative fertility	Standard US population	Expected births
10-14	335	276,837	20,528,072	1.210098361	6.1	6.1	112524.4109	136.1656
15-19	15,343	262,292	20,219,890	58.49587483	292.5	298.5	110835.1145	6483.397
20-24	33,030	274,738	18,964,001	120.2236312	601.1	899.6	103950.9721	12497.36
25-29	32,975	290,046	19,381,336	113.6888631	568.4	1,468.1	106238.5895	12078.14
30-34	25,529	303,023	20,512,388	84.24773037	421.2	1,889.3	112438.4392	9472.683
35-39	11,032	326,552	22,706,664	33.78328719	168.9	2,058.2	124466.34	4204.882
40-44	1,917	320,657	22,441,863	5.978350699	29.9	2,088.1	123014.8361	735.4258
45-54	82	559,312	37,677,952	0.146608691	1.5	2,089.6	206531.2978	30.27928
	120243	2,613,457	182,432,166		2,089.6		1000000	45638.34

(a) (10-14): 1.2, (15-19): 58.5, (20-24): 120.2, (24-29): 113.7,
(30-34): 84.2, (35-39): 33.8, (40-44):6.0, (45 and over):.5;

(b) 2089.6

(c) (10-14): 6.1, (15-19): 298.5, (20-24): 899.6, (25-29): 1468.1,
(30-34): 1889.3, (35-39): 2058.2, (40-44): 2088.1, (45 and over): 2089.6

(d) 45.6

14.4.1.

(a) Immaturity ratio: $1997 - \dfrac{504}{6927} * 100 = 7.3, 2001 - \dfrac{675}{8336} * 100 = 8.1$

(b) Prevalence ratio: Nevada $- \dfrac{430000}{1935000} * 100 = 22.2$, U.S. $- \dfrac{57296000}{279040000} * 100 = 20.5$

(c) Incidence rate $- \dfrac{40758}{281421906} * 100,000 = 14.5$ per 100,000

Chapter 14 Review Exercises

9.

Age (years)	Population[a]	Deaths[b]	U.S. Population[c]	Standard	Death rate	Expected deaths
0-4	566,740	1,178	19,175,798	68138.97	207.8555	141.6306
5-19	1,140,934	224	41,077,577	145964.4	19.63304	28.65724
15-24	1,130,671	954	39,183,891	139235.4	84.37468	117.4794
25-34	1,210,066	1,384	39,891,724	141750.6	114.3739	162.1257
35-44	1,293,741	2,823	45,148,527	160430	218.2044	350.0654
45-54	1,124,305	5,271	37,677,952	133884.2	468.823	627.68
55-64	753,533	8,035	24,274,684	86257.27	1066.31	919.7701
65 and Over	986,115	51,863	34,991,753	124339.1	5259.326	6539.4
Total	8,206,105	71,732	281,421,906	1000000		8886.808

Age-adjusted death rate = $\dfrac{8886.808}{1,000,000} * 1000 = 8.9$

11.

(a) Infant mortality: Total $- \dfrac{1632}{285455}*1000 = 5.7$; White $- \dfrac{957}{182285}*1000 = 5.3$;

Non-White $- \dfrac{675}{103170}*1000 = 6.5$;

(b) Cause of death: Heart disease Total $- \dfrac{57921}{(74636+82776)}*100 = 36.8$;

White $- \dfrac{49624}{(61873+69890)}*100 = 37.7$; Non-White $- \dfrac{8297}{(12763+12886)}*100 = 32.3$

(c) Cancer Total $- \dfrac{37277}{(74636+82776)}*100 = 23.7$; White $- \dfrac{31351}{(61873+69890)}*100 = 23.8$;

Non-White $- \dfrac{5926}{(12763+12886)}*100 = 23.1$

(d) AIDS Total $- \dfrac{2299}{(74636+82776)}*100 = 1.5$; White $- \dfrac{1048}{(61873+69890)}*100 = .8$;

Non-White $- \dfrac{1251}{(12763+12886)}*100 = 4.9$

(e) Immaturity Ratio: Total $- \dfrac{20020}{285455}*100 = 7.0$; White $- \dfrac{12235}{182285}*100 = 6.7$;

Non-White $- \dfrac{7785}{103170}*100 = 7.5$

(f) Incident Rate C-Section: Total $- \dfrac{64424}{285455}*100 = 22.6$; White $- \dfrac{45577}{182285}*100 = 25.0$;

Non-White $- \dfrac{18847}{103170}*100 = 18.3$

13. (a) Crude birth rate: $\dfrac{110{,}984}{6{,}965{,}539}*1000 = 15.9$

(b) General fertility rate: $\dfrac{110{,}984}{2{,}151{,}579}*1000 = 51.6$